PREFACE

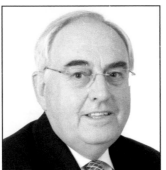

Donald Leeper OBE

The publication of *Design Checks for Public Health Engineering* is a welcome addition to the well received and highly acclaimed *Design Checks for HVAC*, published in 2002.

The design guidance sheets provide information on design inputs, outputs and practical watch points for key building services design topics. It also complements guidance provided in *CIBSE Guide G, Public Health Engineering* and is presented in a format that can be easily incorporated into a firm's quality assurance procedures.

From personal experience I have seen the benefit of such quality procedures. Once embedded within a process information management system, the guidance provides consistent high quality design information. Used for validation and verification, the procedures can also make a key contribution within an overall risk management strategy.

The easy-to-follow layout and the breadth of content makes *Design Checks for Public Health Engineering* a key document for all building services engineers.

Donald Leeper OBE
President, CIBSE 2005-06
Consultant, Zisman Bowyer and Partners LLP

© BSRIA BG2/2006

ACKNOWLEDGEMENTS

BSRIA would like to thank the following sponsors for their contributions to this guide:

Griffiths and Armour Professional Risk
hurleypalmerflatt
Atkins Consultants
Mott MacDonald
Faber Maunsell
EMCOR Group (UK)
Bovis Lend Lease

The project was undertaken under the guidance of an industry steering group. BSRIA would like to thank the following organisations and individuals for their help and guidance:

Zisman Bowyer and Partners LLP
Bovis Lend Lease Ltd
Troup Bywaters Anders
Griffiths and Armour Professional Risk
EMCOR Group (UK) plc
Newham College
Mott MacDonald Ltd
NG Bailey
AMEC
Buro Happold Ltd
Constructing Excellence
Atkins Consultants Ltd
Building LifePlans
Lorien plc
Faber Maunsell
hurleypalmerflatt
CIBSE

Chris Northey
Colin Gibson
David Arnold
Ewan MacGregor
Gary Leek
Gary Mann
Ian Twydell
John Redmond
Keith Williams
Mike Best
Nigel Finn
Peter Jefferson
Peter Mayer
Rudy Menzhausen
Steve Sawers
Vic Jackson
Gay Lawrence Race

The author sought to incorporate the views of the steering group but final editorial control of this document rested with BSRIA.

©BSRIA BG 2/2006   March 2006   ISBN 0 86022 659X   Printed by Multiplex Medway Ltd

OVERVIEW OF DESIGN CHECK TOPICS

Design considerations

1. Design margins
2. Future needs
3. Plant space allowance
4. Spatial co-ordination
5. Maintenance
6. Whole life costing
7. Health and safety

Design issues

8. Site location factors
9. Local authority requirement and discharge consents
10. Mains water availability
11. Contamination prevention
12. Water conservation

Calculations

13. Computer calculations
14. Pipe sizing – cold and hot water services
15. Pipe sizing – above ground sanitary pipework
16. Foul water – below ground drainage systems

Systems and equipment

17. Cold water storage and distribution
18. Hot water storage and distribution
19. Legionnaires' disease – cold water services
20. Legionnaires' disease – hot water services
21. Pressure boosting of water
22. Drinking water systems
23. Water treatment
24. Sanitary accommodation required
25. Drainage systems – above ground foul drainage
26. Foul water – below ground drainage systems
27. Commercial kitchen drainage
28. Surface water – below ground drainage systems
29. Roof drainage
30. Sustainable urban drainage systems
31. Reclaimed water systems – general
32. Reclaimed water systems – greywater
33. Reclaimed water systems – rainwater
34. Piped services
35. Fire systems – water supply

References, bibliography and glossary

INTRODUCTION

Aim

The aim of *Design Checks for Public Health Engineering* is to improve the quality control and performance of the technical design process within the building services industry. The application of best practice should reduce the risk of design errors and omissions and improve the overall efficiency of the design process.

A comprehensive review of current public health engineering design practice and procedures was carried out by BSRIA in consultation with industry. The aim was to identify best practice and current problems, and explore relevant design tools. The resulting good practice guidance for public health engineering design procedures and design management includes:

- A map of the public health engineering design process
- design guidance sheets giving information and guidance on design inputs, outputs and practical watchpoints for a range of key design topics, to aid the design process and reduce errors
- design check sheets which can be included in project quality assurance procedures.

The guidance provides a formal framework to record and review design inputs and encourages designers to consider the requirements for the installation, commissioning, operation and control and subsequent maintenance of their selected systems.

This should lead to improvements in both the design process and in the subsequent implementation of that design, and reduce the risk of problems occurring during installation, commissioning or system operation.

This practical easy to follow guidance can be incorporated into company quality assurance systems to become part of the daily routine of design and can be used to demonstrate compliance with the relevant requirements of *ISO 9001:2000*[i] and *BS 7000 Pt 4:1996*[ii].

The guidance incorporates practical design watchpoints based on feedback from practising engineers and others experienced in design. These vary from avoidance of possible errors or misunderstandings that could be made by inexperienced, junior engineers to very practical tips based on experience of installation, commissioning, and maintenance and facilities management over many years. Use of the *Design Checks for Public Health Engineering* will allow these lessons to be passed on to other engineers, particularly junior engineers, and people working on future projects. This can help improve design quality, reduce risk and increase client confidence.

Note that each area of design guidance addresses sustainability issues where relevant. References to regulations, standards and industry guidance were current at the time of publication. It is advisable to check for updates and additions.

Intended users

This guidance is intended for practising public health design engineers. Clients, professional indemnity insurance providers and others involved in the design process and its outcomes are also potential users. The guidance complements *CIBSE Guide G – Public Health Engineering* and the *Institute of Plumbing and Heating Engineering Plumbing Engineering Services Design Guide* along with other industry guidance (see references and bibliography section).

The check sheets and design inputs and outputs guidance are intended for use by all design engineers, whether to gather information and complete the sheets or to check or sign off as completed. While the more detailed guidance in the design watchpoints is obviously directly useful for junior engineers, experienced engineers will also find it useful when designing a less-familiar system.

Companies may also use the guidance to support formal design quality assurance procedures. The check sheets may be photocopied and are also available, for purchase in electronic format, thus enabling them to be customised for particular projects and kept on specific project files.

Clients should consider this guidance as an indication of good design practice but should not make adherence to it a contractual obligation. Compliance with the guide in itself is not intended to show that the designer has complied with his contractual obligations.

Designers are also suggested to consider alternative designs, methods of working, materials and equipment with the same rigour as their own design and this guidance can help in that process.

THE CASE FOR QUALITY CONTROL

Good design is central to the achievement of quality buildings that satisfy client requirements, yet all too often defects and failures that occur after occupation can be shown to have their origin in design deficiencies. It has been shown that 50% of claims notified to PII insurers come from matters arising during the design stage of a project with 21% of these being attributed to building services elements and 11% being attributed to public health systems. [iii]

Many quality assurance schemes are primarily concerned with general design management and the logging of project decisions, rather than the actual quality of the design itself. As there is no industry standard that assures technical design quality, and therefore no procedures for designers and clients to follow, both parties can be exposed to risk. Design procedures should meet adequate quality standards such as *BS 7000 Pt4:1996*[ii] and be adequately checked, but there is insufficient guidance on how to do this for building services design. This publication meets the need for procedures which can be adopted across the industry.

More fundamentally, problems and errors can recur over many projects, with the same mistakes being repeated. An individual engineer may have learnt from experience, but that learning is often not passed on to others. Even if a solution to an error or problem is found during a construction project, the cause of the initial problem may often not be recorded at all. Subsequent projects involving the same company may see errors repeated.

Ways to capture information effectively in a no-blame context need to be implemented for learning to be effectively transmitted not just within one organisation or one project but also across many projects and organisations. This guidance enables organisations to better implement technical design checks as part of their quality assurance process and to meet the relevant requirements of *ISO 9001:2000*[i] and *BS 7000 Part 4:1996*[ii]. It can also encourage design organisations to add to the design watchpoints to provide further dissemination of lessons learnt within the organisation.

Design errors - examples and case studies

Problems that have their origin in design vary from minor omissions to major errors. Some are not realised until the building has been operational for some while. Others may be identified in time to make changes or remedy the situation prior to handover, such as recognised during a design review, at contract award stage, during installation or during the commissioning process. Although these errors can be remedied prior to occupation this is effectively fire-fighting not fire prevention, and is certainly not ideal. Design errors and omissions should be prevented or identified during the design process. Any design errors identified subsequently will be costly in time and rework. The firm held responsible for these problems will risk a loss of reputation and increased PII premiums.

Specific examples of design errors and issues which should be considered during design and which could lead to operational problems or subsequent litigation, include:

- Repeated blockages and flooding from foul drains and soil stacks
- Failure to allow adequate access around plant items for maintenance
- Insufficient hot and cold water storage capacities
- Incorrectly sized pipework
- Excessive noise from pipework
- Insufficient pipe thermal insulation leading to energy waste and/or risk of freezing
- Insufficient pressure boosting of internal water supply
- Presence of pipework deadlegs resulting in a risk of legionnaires' disease
- Insufficient hydraulic capacity for drainage systems
- Incorrectly sized and installed commercial kitchen grease separators
- Non-compliance with *The Water Supply (Water Fittings) Regulations* resulting in a risk of water contamination
- Incorrectly identified pipework for reclaimed water systems resulting in a water contamination risk
- Thermostatic mixing valves not specified for applications where occupants are vulnerable to scalding
- Flooding from roof-valley gutters and surface-water drains
- Rodent and insect problems
- Cross infections and bad odours.

Many design errors can be remedied without recourse to litigation although there will be cost penalties. The following case studies illustrate design errors that have occurred in practice. Use of formal design quality assurance procedures and design guidance can help prevent errors and save companies considerable time and cost.

The design guidance and check sheets included in this guide list many watchpoints on operation and control issues, and on access and maintenance issues, and provide a framework to support formal design quality assurance procedures. Their use ought to deliver improved client service and provide a basis for demonstrating that due care has been taken in design.

THE CASE FOR QUALITY CONTROL

Case Study 1

The consultant required a specialist contractor to design a siphonic rainwater disposal system. The resulting system proved to be defective.

The consultant had no previous experience of such a system and could not check its suitability. The consultant had not informed the client that the design had to be carried out by a specialist appointed by the contractor. Even though the consultant was not the designer of the system the consultant was held liable as they had failed to warn the client of a lack of experience resulting in the design being carried out by others.

Lesson learned

All consultants should refer to their contract of appointment to establish the design liability for specialist design work carried out by others and cannot assume that, because it is being designed by others, the consultant will not be liable.

Case Study 2

A petrol interceptor proved to be wrongly sized in a naturally ventilated multi-storey car park as the consultant had not considered the rainfall captured by the exposed top level of the car park.

The consultant, having had experience of designing underground car parks, knew to consider the effects of a sprinkler system on a petrol interceptor but, in the absence of a sprinkler system, had not considered rainfall in an over-ground car park.

Lessons learned

It is wrong to assume that what was required on a previous project (no matter how successful) will be the same as required for the next project. Every design proposal needs to go back to first principles.

© BSRIA BG2/2006

THE CASE FOR QUALITY CONTROL

Case Study 3

The surface water run-off for an urban development was designed to be disposed of through a series of soakaways.

The public health designer had considered the existing ground conditions to be suitable for this purpose but had not reviewed the design when the full extent of the hard landscaping was confirmed.

This resulted in a much increased level of run-off and also changed the characteristics of the ground adjacent to the soakaways. The remedial work was at the cost of the consultant in settlement of the claim.

Lessons learned

Designs need to be constantly reviewed to ensure that any design dependent on the work of others remains adequate when details of that other work becomes known.

PII insurer recommendations

Some professional indemnity insurance providers provide guidance to their clients on good practice to minimise the risk of claims. For example, Griffiths and Armour have published a lessons learned document based on analysis of professional indemnity claims[iv]. This includes recommendations during the design stage to:

- Ensure that a suitably qualified person checks all drawings, documents and calculations
- designers follow in-house quality assurance procedures
- designers consider all alternatives with the same rigour as the original design proposals.

Griffiths and Armour advise that good quality control in the design office, (including crosschecking of related work) is essential to avoid unnecessary design errors. Guidance is also provided on other issues which may arise during the design process, such as advice from other team members, the use of information or drawings prepared by others and the use of computers and innovative design.

THE CASE FOR QUALITY CONTROL

BS EN ISO 9000 series and BS 7000 requirements

The following section provides a brief summary of the relevant sections of the above standards.

BS EN ISO 9000 series

ISO 9000:2000 provides guidance on quality management fundamentals and vocabulary. *ISO 9001:2000*[i], (which cancels and replaces the previous *ISO 9001, 9002* and *9003*) covers the requirements for a quality management system. The main objective of the series is to give purchasers of a product or a service an assurance that the quality of the product and/or service provided by a supplier meets their requirements.

The series of standards defines and sets out a definitive list of features and characteristics which it is considered should be present in an organisation's quality management system through documented policies, manuals and procedures. The overall aim is a systematic approach to quality assurance and control.

Section 4.2 of *ISO 9001:2000*[i] refers to the documentation required for a quality management system, including the need for a quality manual and documented procedures. Section 7 covers product realisation with 7.1 (c) referring to the requirement for verification, validation, monitoring inspection and test activities specific to the product and the criteria for product acceptance.

Section 7.3 addresses design and development. Specific requirements include the need for :

- Design input review and records (7.3.2)
- Design output review and verification (7.3.3)
- Design and development review (7.3.4)
- Design and development verification (7.3.5)
- Design and development validation (7.3.6).

There is a clear requirement to:
- Review and record design inputs and outputs
- verify the design to ensure it can meet the design requirements
- review the design process to identify and remedy potential problems.

ISO 9004:2000[v] complements *ISO 9001* by giving guidance on a wider range of objectives of a quality management system than *ISO 9001*. This is cross-referenced to the sections of *ISO 9001* and focuses in particular on continual performance improvement.

Under Section 7.3.3, suggested design verification activities include alternative design and development calculations and evaluation against lessons learned from previous designs. Suggested design validation activities include the validation of engineering design prior to construction, installation or applications, and validation of software outputs.

BS7000: Design management systems

BS7000 covers design management systems and comprises:

- Part 1: Guide to managing product design
- Part 2: Guide to managing the design of manufactured products
- Part 3: Guide to managing service design
- Part 4: Guide to managing design in construction
- Part 10: Glossary of terms used in design management.

BS 7000 Part 4:1996[ii] is the most relevant of the *BS7000* parts as it is specifically directed toward management of the design process within the construction industry for all organisations and for all types of construction project.

Section 4 specifically covers design process management including the responsibilities of the design leader, the design brief and the specific design stages and procedures including design change control and design documentation.

Design procedures are covered in Section 4.7 with design input (4.7.3), design process (4.7.4) and design output (4.7.5) separately identified. The Standard states that formal procedures should be used for all projects, with design procedures clearly recorded and relevant design criteria and constraints listed. All design inputs should be validated and all design outputs should be subject to a stated verification strategy. To allow traceability, significant design assumptions and decisions should be recorded as the design proceeds.

Annex A provides information on validation and verification and states that a risk assessment exercise can be conducted. It also points out the importance of the cost of increased rigour against the risk of an increased penalty. The Standard states that all design methods and sources of design data should be validated.

The use of the design checks guidance

The design checks guidance can be used to assist with compliance with the above standards as part of a quality assurance scheme, as it provides a formal method of recording and checking design inputs and outputs within a quality control framework. By asking for cross-referencing and data sources, the design checks will assist with validation of design inputs, while relevant watchpoints and key design checks can assist the verification of design outputs.

THE PUBLIC HEALTH ENGINEERING DESIGN PROCESS

Design is a complex process which involves translating ideas, proposals and statements of needs and requirements into precise descriptions of a specific product(s)[vi]. Design problems are often ill-defined, their solutions often not self-evident. Designers try to achieve a solution that is satisfactory or appropriate. There is rarely one correct answer to a design problem, different designers might arrive at different but possibly equally satisfactory solutions.

Two major features characterise the design process. First, design tends to evolve through a series of stages at which the solution is increasingly designed at greater levels of detail, moving from broad outline through to fine detail. Second, design tends to contain iterative cycles of activities during which designs, or design components, are continually trialled, tested, evaluated and refined. Feedback loops are therefore an essential component of design. Most models of the design process therefore involve many feedback and iteration loops; even some simple ones use a spiral model to illustrate the process.

Design within construction increasingly involves a number of interdependent professional disciplines with concurrent design processes. It is invariably iterative. Although design may originate with a client need and then a design brief, the design brief itself is not a finite object and often evolves during the design process. In practice, the design process involves constant communication and clarification between team members, with many design steps being revisited as the design evolves and develops. This is recognised to some extent with the standard process stages of outline design, scheme design and further/detail design.[vii] There are a number of models of the building process, most of which show this as a largely linear process, ranging from the stages in the RIBA Plan of Work to the Generic Design and Construction Process Protocol developed by Salford University[viii]. This breaks the design and construction process down into ten distinct phases which are grouped into four broad stages: pre-project, pre-construction, construction and post-completion.

However, none of the commonly-used models show the design part of the process in detail, let alone the building services design process. One of the tasks proposed for this guide was to model the building services design process in order to provide relevant guidance and show the various design tasks that form part of the process in context. This proved to be very complex. If the integral iterative and feedback loops are included, the model effectively needs to be three dimensional (if not four, with addition of a time element), as it is not possible to represent it clearly in two dimensions.

In the event, a detailed analysis of design procedures and tasks was carried out for building services design. After considerable research and consultation with industry a model was successfully developed that departs from the evolutionary model of design, where design proceeds through a series of stages from broad outline through to fine detail. Instead, a simple linear model was proposed that is much closer to a pure design process. This provides a single design sequence, from statement of need, through problem analysis, synthesis and evaluation to final solution. This enables design tasks to be clearly linked to both preceding and succeeding actions.

The building services design process was mapped both as a sequence of design tasks and as a series of topics that make up the design process. This provides an overview of the design process to both inform the designer and enable design elements to be seen in context.

For simplicity, the processes set out in this guide are therefore presented as a sequential, linear flow. In practice, there will be overlap from one stage to another, and it may be necessary to revise calculations or modify assumptions at almost any stage. This may in turn lead to a series of knock-on revisions. These have associated cost implications which should also be considered in managing and controlling the overall process.

The design process

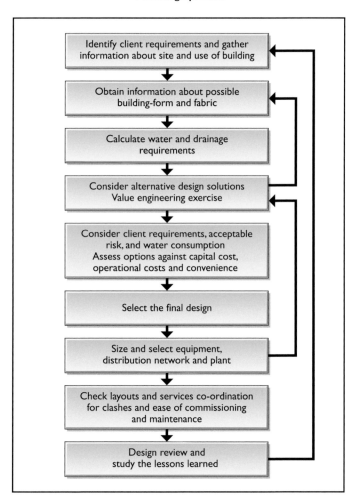

THE PUBLIC HEALTH ENGINEERING DESIGN PROCESS

Public health engineering design tasks and design map

The flow chart below shows a very simplified, linear version of the main public health engineering design tasks. Some primary feedback loops are shown, but in practice there are often feedback loops between all tasks and even within specific tasks.

This sequence of design tasks was then linked to the detail of the design process and the various design choices and considerations in order to develop a design map. This is shown in the form of an Ishikawa or fishbone diagram, starting from client need on the left with various branches feeding into the main design line to eventually reach design completion. An essential part of this design process is the need for design feedback to inform future projects.

A simplified map is shown below and the full detailed design map for the public health engineering design process is provided as a fold-out inside the back cover.

As previously explained, the map presents a linear view of design, with iteration and intermediate feedback omitted. The main branches feed into a central spine in the approximate sequence of design output.

The individual branches and sub-branches show relevant design topics which can be related to specific design guidance sheets. Some simplifications or expansions have been made for clarity. In practice, many design tasks would be carried out concurrently but the map illustrates an approximate design sequence.

Although the map inevitably simplifies what is a very complex design process, it does provide an overview of the public health engineering design process to inform both designer and client. It can also show the effects of early assumptions or late changes on the design process, such as the amount of design assumptions that have to be made if a design task such as plant sizing were carried out at an initial stage in the project. Equally the effects of a late client change on design rework will be clearly visible for example where there is a change to occupancy, or to future needs when the design has already reached the stage of system selection and detailed sizing and layout.

A simplified design process map

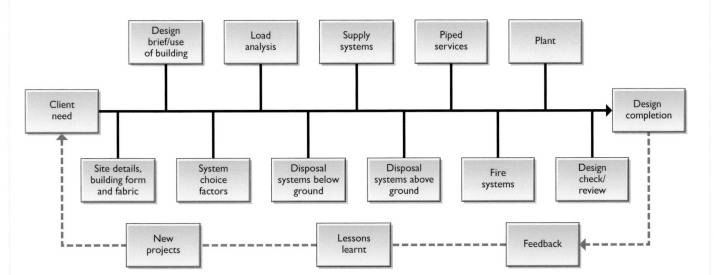

OVERVIEW OF DESIGN GUIDE SECTIONS

The guidance is organised into four sections covering a range of topics relevant to public health engineering:

Design considerations

This section covers the key topics relevant to client requirements and services strategy to be considered at design inception, such as ownership of land, ownership of service, future needs, design margins and plant space allowance. It also covers issues that relate to the whole design concept such as whole-life costing, spatial co-ordination and consideration of maintenance requirements.

Design issues

This section covers the key topics relevant to analysis and definition of the client brief and client requirements to determine information on the site and use of the building. This includes site location factors, mains water availability and contamination prevention.

Calculations

This section covers the key base calculations used for public health engineering design, including pipework and drainage sizing, together with an overview of the use of computer design packages.

Systems and equipment

This section covers the main systems and equipment items for public health engineering design such as cisterns and calorifiers, water treatment equipment, sanitary accommodation and drainage systems.

Design considerations inform the whole design process, with the other sections following the approximate design sequence used in practice, as shown in the diagram opposite.

For each topic the guidance provides two pages with a check sheet on the left hand page and a design guidance sheet on the right as shown on the opposite page.

Design guidance sheets

The design guidance sheet provides design inputs, design information, design outputs, key design checks and design watchpoints.

Design inputs

The technical input required for the design or selection of that particular design item such as required pressure, water demand and design temperatures.

Design information

Design information which is necessary for design decisions, system layouts or selection of equipment such as the building plans location of fittings, available space for plant, type and use of building.

Design outputs

The required design output from that particular part of the design process to either inform future design or to form part of the specification or design production, such as schematic diagrams, system layout drawings, schedules of equipment sizes and duties.

Key design checks

Key design checks are those points to particularly check as part of the design process.

Design watchpoints

These provide guidance to inform the design process as a series of check-points or items to be aware of during the design. The watchpoints are grouped together in three to four linked sections to show that design decisions affect not only on the sizing and selection of systems, but also on installation, commissionability, future operation and control, maintainability, and capital and operating costs.

The watchpoints are based on the collected experience of many practising design engineers, but should not be taken to be an exhaustive or definitive list of everything to be considered. Every design project is different and has differing needs, and it is the responsibility of the design engineer to consider fully all the design requirements. Design engineers and design practices should be encouraged to add their own additional watchpoints and add to the pool of feedback knowledge to inform further design projects.

Design check sheets

The design check sheet can be used as part of a quality assurance system to provide a formal record of inputs and outputs from different design stages, cross-referenced to the design file. This will facilitate compliance with the requirements of the quality assurance system and of *ISO 9001* as well as enabling a clear record to be kept of design progress and design information.

Example of the design sequence used in practice

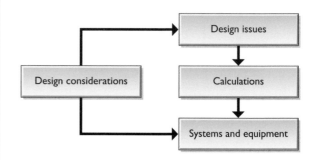

OVERVIEW OF DESIGN GUIDE SECTIONS

The **design inputs and outputs** from the guidance sheet for each topic are reproduced here and can be checked off and cross-referenced to data sources, thus allowing easy tracking of design information in the case of design changes or queries.

Key design checks are reproduced to encourage designers to continually check and review their design. Space is also allowed for **project specific checks and notes**. No design guidance manual can be fully comprehensive for all design applications, therefore it is the responsibility of the designer to add additional information as required by a particular project.

Use of design checks guidance

This design guidance is intended to inform the design process and provide detail to aid the designer. It does not cover the relative merits of different system or equipment choices, but provides guidance that will, for example, help engineers to design the selected system(s) after the initial design strategy has been agreed.

A design project is likely to refer to many of the guidance sheets during the design process. The example overleaf shows the sheets that may be relevant to the design of cold water storage and distribution.

References and bibliography

A references and bibliography section at the end of this guide provides reference to additional guidance that covers both general design issues and specific references that are relevant to the individual design topics.

Sample design check and design guidance page

OVERVIEW OF DESIGN GUIDE SECTIONS

Example of guide use for a cold water storage and distribution system, showing relevant topics

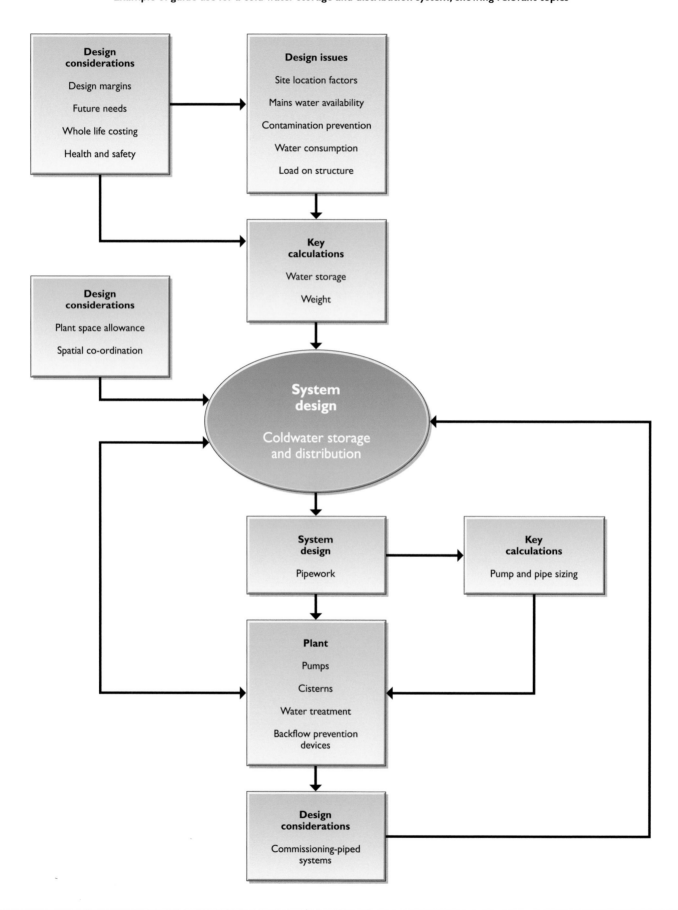

© BSRIA BG2/2006

DESIGN CONSIDERATIONS

1   DESIGN MARGINS

Project title.. **Project No**................................. **Design stage**...................

Engineer.. **Revision No**.............................. **Date**...........................

Checked by.. **Approved by** .... **Date**...........................

Design Information

- Client brief including future needs requirements and any specific requirements for system or plant duplication or critical systems

- Details of building and space use to determine the required level of system reliability

✓ **Notes / Design file cross-reference**

❑

❑

Design outputs

- Overall design margin strategy, including quality assurance procedures, and design reviews

- Clear identification in the design file of any margins used within design calculations, together with a written justification for their use

- Clear statement of operating limits of the design for the client

✓ **Notes / Design file cross-reference**

❑

❑

❑

Key design checks

- Agree design margin policy with the client as part of a value engineering strategy

- At the end of a calculation procedure, review all margins used to avoid possible double counting and remove excess margins

- At the design review stage, review again the appropriateness of any design margins used

✓ **Notes / Design file cross-reference**

❑

❑

❑

Project specific checks and notes

✓ **Notes / Design file cross-reference**

❑

❑

❑

I   DESIGN MARGINS

Why consider this?

- Avoidance of unnecessary oversizing of plant and systems
- Client future needs
- Equipment and space selection
- Plant space allowance

Design information

- Client brief including future needs requirements and any specific requirements for system or plant duplication or critical systems
- Details of building and space use to determine the required level of system reliability

See also: Future Needs

Design outputs

- Overall design margin strategy, including quality assurance procedures, and design reviews
- Clear identification in the design file of any margins used within design calculations, together with a written justification for their use
- Clear statement of operating limits of the design for the client

Key design checks

- Agree design margin policy with the client as part of a value engineering strategy
- At the end of a calculation procedure, review all margins used to avoid possible double counting and remove excess margins
- At the design review stage, review again the appropriateness of any design margins used

DESIGN WATCHPOINTS

General watchpoints

1. Clearly identify and justify the use of all margins added during the design process in the design file.
2. Reduce the need for margins where possible. Provide the client with a clear statement of operating limits of the design to ensure that the client is aware of, and satisfied with, the anticipated performance of the system.
3. Clarify with the client the required level of system reliability. Critical systems and services will require a different level of safety provided by redundancy, or installed plant margins, to non-critical ones.
4. At the end of a calculation procedure, review all margins used to avoid possible double counting and remove excess margins.
5. At the design review stage, review again the appropriateness of any design margins used.
6. Design margins can be added for legitimate operational reasons and these should be clearly identified.
7. Margins are sometimes added to allow for design or installation uncertainties and missing design information. Uncertainties or assumptions should be clearly flagged and reviewed when correct information is available. Reduce uncertainties in the design as much as possible by clarifying the brief.
8. Designers should always ensure that their reasonable design margins are retained when considering value engineering and cost saving alternatives.

Installation, operation and control

9. Margins added to pipework systems to account for future needs can result in low initial operating fluid-velocities.

Economics

10. Agree the margins policy with the client as part of a value engineering strategy.
11. Sizing systems and equipment for anticipated future expansion can result in lower operating efficiencies and higher running costs. Allow space for future plant items.
12. Where a known margin is to be applied to a system to cater for future expansion, consider selecting plant and equipment that can provide a variable supply, such as variable speed pumps.
13. Applying margins to a system can lead to increased installation costs as well as increased capital costs.

© BSRIA BG2/2006

2   FUTURE NEEDS

Project title.. **Project No**... **Design stage**..................

Engineer... **Revision No**... **Date**................................

Checked by... **Approved by**.. **Date**................................

Design information

- Client statement of anticipated future needs requirements

Notes / Design file cross-reference

Design outputs

- Input to the client brief on the need for flexibility and client requirements for future change

- Agreed design strategy for future needs

- Information for the client on the implications of the adopted design, in terms of performance and costs

- Implementation strategy to provide client with contingency plans for possible future changes

Notes / Design file cross-reference

Key design checks

- Agree the client requirements for future flexibility at the briefing stage

- Consider the capacity and location of load bearing areas within the building in relation to possible future changes

- Do not automatically add over-capacity to all plant at the initial design stage as a solution to future flexibility

Notes / Design file cross-reference

Project specific checks and notes

Notes / Design file cross-reference

2 FUTURE NEEDS

Why consider this?

Consideration of future needs at the design stage is essential for:

- Future flexibility. Organisational change can result in changes of occupancy density, occupancy hours and building use
- Future expansion

Design information

- Client statement of anticipated future needs requirements

See also: Design Margins

Design outputs

- Input to the client brief on the need for flexibility and client requirements for future change
- Agreed design strategy for future needs
- Information for the client on the implications of the adopted design, in terms of performance and costs
- Implementation strategy to provide the client with contingency plans for possible future changes

Key design checks

- Agree the client requirements for future flexibility at the briefing stage
- Consider the capacity and location of load bearing areas within the building in relation to possible future changes
- Do not automatically add over-capacity to all plant at the initial design stage as a solution to future flexibility

DESIGN WATCHPOINTS

General watchpoints

1. Discuss the use of the building and types of possible future change with the client as early as possible, including the facilities management team
2. All team members need to be aware of the policy for future needs permitting due allowances in space and structure to be incorporated in the design.
3. As a project progresses, the scope for specifying flexible public health services reduces, with a consequent increase in the associated cost. Flexible services design should ideally be considered during the project definition design phase and further developed during the outline proposal stage.
4. Liase with the architect and structural designers to check that the building structure does not restrict future changes.
5. At an early stage check the capability of incoming utility supplies to satisfy projected future needs.
6. Allow adequate distribution space for additional future systems and equipment that may be required as identified in a future needs strategy, for example check that risers have sufficient capacity for planned additional services.
7. Consider the introduction of soft spots in the building structure to allow provision of future services risers.
8. Location of holes in the structural frame should be considered at an early stage.
9. Allow adequate plant space for any future plant that may be required as identified in a future needs strategy.
10. Consider the capacity and location of load-bearing areas within the building in relation to possible future increases in services plant.

11. Do not automatically add over-capacity to all plant at the initial design stage as a solution to future flexibility. Design with over-capacity only where it is too expensive or difficult to add in latter. If over-capacity is included check that plant can operate efficiently at normal operating conditions.
12. Sizing systems and equipment for anticipated future expansion can result in lower operating efficiencies and increased running costs.
13. Consider the future needs for provision of below-ground drainage at an early stage, such as for future kitchen or laboratory provision.
14. Consider designing systems for anticipated future maximum occupancy.
15. Simple designs often allow more scope for future flexibility than complex, or over-specified ones.

Economics

16. Designing in flexibility can save considerable future expense.
17. Consider the use of prefabricated, modular services and control systems as these can facilitate quick and cost effective change.
18. Different design options should be assessed on a whole-life costing basis and tested against the design brief.

3   PLANT SPACE ALLOWANCE

Project title .... **Project No**. .... **Design stage** ....

Engineer .... **Revision No** .... **Date** ....

Checked by .... **Approved by** .... **Date** ....

Design information

	✓	Notes / Design file cross-reference
• Preliminary architectural layout drawings	☐	
• Required plant loads, fire protection and ventilation requirements	☐	
• Manufacturers' equipment data for proposed plant for accurate plant dimensions	☐	
• Maintenance data for plant items, such as frequency, tasks, and access requirements	☐	
• Details of building use and future need requirements	☐	
• Position of services risers and sizes	☐	
• Structural design layouts	☐	
• Loading imposed by heavy plant and storage tanks	☐	
• Levels	☐	
• Services co-ordination	☐	
• Location and size of water storage tanks	☐	

Design outputs

	✓	Notes / Design file cross-reference
• Sufficient information to enable a planning application to be made	☐	
• Drawings providing dimensioned plant space requirements, leading to co-ordinated detailed plant room layouts encompassing all services	☐	
• Structural load information for structural engineers	☐	

Key design checks

	✓	Notes / Design file cross-reference
• Check client requirements for future needs	☐	
• Check building use and any need for standby or duplicate plant	☐	
• Check location is suitable for access and maintenance needs	☐	

3 PLANT SPACE ALLOWANCE

Project title.. **Project No**.......................... **Design stage**................

Engineer.. **Revision No**........................ **Date**..............................

Checked by.. **Approved by**...................... **Date**..............................

Key design checks (cont.)

✓ **Notes / Design file cross-reference**

- Allow adequate space for installation, access, maintenance and plant replacement ☐

- Consider acoustic requirements and required noise control measures ☐

- Provide the structural engineers with details of plant operating weights so that the roof and other supporting structures can be designed accordingly ☐

Project specific checks and notes

✓ **Notes / Design file cross-reference**

☐

☐

☐

3 PLANT SPACE ALLOWANCE

Why consider this?

- Building configuration
- Determination of required access and egress routes
- Maintenance requirements
- Structural design

Design information

- Preliminary architectural layout drawings
- Required plant loads, fire protection and ventilation requirements
- Manufacturers' equipment data for proposed plant for accurate plant dimensions
- Maintenance data for plant items, such as frequency, tasks and access requirements
- Details of building use and future need requirements
- Position of services risers and sizes
- Structural design layouts
- Loading imposed by heavy plant and storage tanks
- Levels
- Services co-ordination
- Location and size of water storage tanks

Design outputs

- Sufficient information to enable a planning application to be made
- Drawings providing dimensioned plant space requirements, leading to co-ordinated detailed plant room layouts encompassing all services
- Structural load information for structural engineers

Key design checks

- Check client requirements for future needs
- Check building use and any need for standby or duplicate plant
- Check location is suitable for access and maintenance needs
- Allow adequate space for installation, access, maintenance and plant replacement
- Consider acoustic requirements and required noise control measures
- Provide the structural engineers with details of plant operating weights so that roofs and other support structures can be designed accordingly

See also: Spatial Co-ordination

DESIGN WATCHPOINTS

General watchpoints

1. Plant space requirements must be considered at an early stage in design as services can occupy a large percentage of the building volume. The key factors in planning the space for services are size, weight, location and relationship.
2. Check client requirements for future needs.
3. Check building use and any requirements for standby or duplicate plant.
4. Allow adequate space for getting the plant in and out of the building, for both new build and replacement. Consider whether access for cranes will be required, or if side panels of high level plant rooms will need to be removed.
5. Comply with relevant regulations, such as *CDM, Means of Escape,* and *Health and Safety at Work.*
6. Allow sufficient space to comply with any supply authority access and maintenance requirements for their equipment.
7. Locate plant where it is accessible by the appropriate authorities.
8. Provide the structural engineer with weight details of plant, including pipework, so the structures can be designed accordingly. This is particularly important for roof plant. Always use operating weight and not shipping or dry weight as some plant can increase in weight substantially when filled with fluids such as water.
9. Ideally, plant rooms should be well proportioned and square or rectangular to maximise space efficiency and flexibility. Internal columns within the room can significantly reduce available space.
10. Locate plant as closely as possible to the centre of the area it serves. This will reduce losses and take up less space *en route.*
11. Allow sufficient space for connections to plant. This includes smaller items such as pumps. Turning radii for large diameter pipework can be considerable.
12. Try to locate plant so that associated pipework services can enter and exit the plant space where required. This will save space within the plant room.
13. Consider acoustic requirements and allow sufficient space for proper noise control, both to prevent break-out noise and to allow for proper vibration control.

Installation, operation and control

14. Allow adequate working space for plant installation.

Access and maintenance

15. Provide adequate means of escape from plant rooms. Evacuation and escape routes through plant areas should be kept clear.
16. Check that access is sufficient to allow removal and replacement of the largest plant item.
17. Check that the location is suitable for access and maintenance needs and that plant room height is sufficient for safe access and maintenance.
18. In some instances, the same maintenance space allowance can be used for adjacent items of plant, assuming that maintenance is not carried out on both simultaneously.
19. Consider the positioning of items of plant, filters and strainers when laying out plant rooms to make access easier.
20. Be careful not to impinge on maintenance space when laying pipework services.

Economics

21. Building space costs money and oversized plantrooms can incur criticism from clients and cost controllers. However, too little space will make maintenance more difficult, expensive and less likely to happen. Careful consideration of plant and maintenance requirements and health and safety requirements is therefore needed.

4   SPATIAL CO-ORDINATION

Project title... **Project No**.......................... **Design stage**..............

Engineer.. **Revision No**........................ **Date**..........................

Checked by... **Approved by**...................... **Date**..........................

Design information

✓ **Notes / Design file cross-reference**

- Architectural drawings, including layouts, sections, elevations and construction details ☐
- Structural frame details such as positions of beams and columns ☐
- Details of other services to be installed ☐
- Requirements of the *CDM Regulations* ☐
- Fire compartmentation details ☐

Design outputs

✓ **Notes / Design file cross-reference**

- Information for the rest of the design team to assist scheme design layouts ☐
- Input to co-ordinated detailed design drawings ☐
- Information for the rest of the design team to assist scheme design layouts ☐

Key design checks

✓ **Notes / Design file cross-reference**

- Identify and resolve potential clash points ☐
- Inform architects and other team members of access and space requirements ☐
- Consider each space and all visible items; agree architectural specification ☐
- Allow sufficient space for the falls required on drainage systems ☐

Project specific checks and notes

✓ **Notes / Design file cross-reference**

☐
☐
☐

4   SPATIAL CO-ORDINATION

Essential for

- Detailed plant and services layout drawings
- Avoidance of clashes, installation problems and re-design
- Safe and easy access to plant and equipment

Design information

- Architectural drawings, including layouts, sections, elevations and construction details
- Structural frame details such as positions of beams and columns
- Details of other services to be installed
- Requirements of the *CDM Regulations*
- Fire compartmentation details

See also: Design Margins, Future Needs, Plant Space Allowance

Design outputs

- Information for the rest of the design team to assist scheme design layouts
- Input to co-ordinated detailed design drawings
- Information for the rest of the design team to assist scheme design layouts

Key design checks

- Identify and resolve potential clash points
- Inform architects and other team members of access and space requirements
- Consider each space and all visible items; agree architectural specification
- Allow sufficient space for the falls required on drainage systems

DESIGN WATCHPOINTS

General watchpoints

1. A full knowledge of all the services systems being installed is required so that effective co-ordination of the design and layout can be carried out. Potential clash points need to be identified and resolved. Changes on site are inevitably more disruptive and expensive than alterations during the design stage.

2. The allocation of responsibilities between the consultant and contractor for co-ordination information should be clearly defined.

3. Work to the building grid pattern for locating equipment where possible.

4. Allow adequate space for all equipment.

5. Adequate space for maintaining means of escape and evacuation routes should be provided when space layouts are being determined.

6. Allow sufficient space for the falls required on pipework systems, particularly drainage.

7. Allow sufficient space for pipework fittings. Turning radii on large size pipework can be considerable.

8. Check that adequate drainage is provided. Drainage points are required in all areas where water is stored (such as in cisterns and tank rooms) to facilitate drain down for cleaning or in the case of a leak.

Installation, operation and control

9. Check that all builders work requirements have been clearly communicated to the project team.

10. Check that the building structure permits required penetrations.

11. When preparing builders work schedules for penetrations through the fabric, check that the holes asked for are sufficient for services to be installed rather than just house them. This may mean a hole substantially larger than the pipe passing through it, as the service needs to be manoeuvred through the opening. It may also have flanges and insulation.

12. Check that where services penetrate walls and floors (fire rated or not) that they are correctly detailed.

13. Allow sufficient space to install pipework fittings, remembering to allow for insulation thickness. Valves need adequate space to be fitted.

Access and maintenance

14. Inform architects and other design team members of access requirements, for example by issuing marked up drawings. Access requirements should be agreed and included in specifications.

15. Check there is adequate access in and around the site for installation, maintenance and deliveries for services. Make the project manager aware of requirements at an early stage.

16. Allow sufficient space for access for commissioning and maintenance of pipework and ductwork fittings. Check manufacturers' guidelines for access space.

17. Allow adequate space for plant and equipment replacement.

18. Avoid joints in distribution systems in locations that are inaccessible, or difficult to access.

19. Provide access ladders, platforms or walkways where necessary where plant cannot be reached by stepladders. Provide step-overs to pipework where required.

20. Co-ordination of risers and service voids should consider installation sequence, support requirements, pipework falls and component access requirements.

Economics

21. Consider the issues surrounding central and/or local plant to achieve optimum performance and best use of space, for example in a remote room it may be more beneficial to provide a local hot water heater rather than run hot water services from the central plant.

5   MAINTENANCE

Project title.. **Project No**.............................. **Design stage**...................

Engineer.. **Revision No**........................... **Date**.................................

Checked by... **Approved by**......................... **Date**.................................

Design information

✓ **Notes / Design file cross-reference**

- Details of client maintenance policy ☐

- Architectural drawings including layouts and sections ☐

- Information on services to be installed ☐

- Evacuation and means of escape routes through plant areas so maintenance tasks will not restrict movement in an emergency ☐

- Access in and around the site for maintenance equipment and deliveries ☐

Design outputs

✓ **Notes / Design file cross-reference**

- Operation and maintenance strategy for the public health services systems ☐

- Specific system and equipment maintenance requirements in operation and maintenance manuals ☐

- The effect on detailed system design drawings and specification ☐

Key design checks

✓ **Notes / Design file cross-reference**

- Check compliance with the *CDM Regulations* ☐

- Check the purpose of the building to determine the level of maintenance required. Critical systems and services will require a different level of maintenance to non-critical ones ☐

- Check that standard design guidance is followed regarding provision of maintenance equipment on all systems ☐

- Check the time period for availability of spares ☐

- Check ease of obtaining spares ☐

Project specific checks and notes

✓ **Notes / Design file cross-reference**

☐
☐
☐

© BSRIA BG2/2006

5 MAINTENANCE

Why consider this?

Consideration of the maintenance requirements of public health systems at the design stage is essential for:

- Correct equipment and system selection and layout
- Safe access to facilities
- Adequate plant space allowance
- Future commissioning of systems
- Operation and maintenance of systems
- Consideration of whole life costs
- Risk assessment and *CDM Regulations* documentation

Design information

- Details of client maintenance policy
- Architectural drawings including layouts and sections
- Information on services to be installed
- Evacuation and means of escape routes through plant areas so maintenance tasks will not restrict movement in an emergency
- Access in and around the site for maintenance equipment and deliveries

Design outputs

- Operation and maintenance strategy for the public health services systems
- Specific system and equipment maintenance requirements in operation and maintenance manuals
- The effect on detailed system design drawings and specification

Key design checks

- Check compliance with the *CDM Regulations*
- Check the purpose of the building to determine the level of maintenance required. Critical systems and services will require a different level of maintenance to non-critical ones
- Check that standard design guidance is followed regarding provision of maintenance equipment on all systems
- Check the time period for availability of spares
- Check ease of obtaining spares

See also: Spatial Co-ordination, Whole Life Costing

DESIGN WATCHPOINTS

General watchpoints

1. If applicable, consult with the facilities management team at an early stage if possible.

2. The plant and systems must be arranged and located to permit adequate access for maintenance without exposing the maintenance staff to undue risk. This is a requirement of the *Construction Design and Management (CDM) Regulations*.

3. Design with maintenance in mind. Consider the positioning of items of plant when laying out plant rooms to make access easier and maintenance simple, and allow adequate space around all plant items. If an item that requires maintenance is hard to reach, it will tend to be maintained less well.

4. Design simple, straightforward systems where possible. Complicated systems generally require more maintenance.

5. Consider both current and proposed legislation that may affect maintenance.

6. Try to use standard arrangements wherever possible so that the same spare parts can be used on a number of systems and components. This reduces the amount of spares that need to be kept, and also improves reliability through interchangeability.

7. Input from the planning supervisor may be required to determine the methodology for maintenance of plant and equipment, for example if some plant is in an awkward location, therefore it may have particular requirements in terms of access and working practices for maintenance.

8. The need for plant to be maintained may have an effect on members of staff and the public. Check whether carrying out maintenance of a particular piece of plant would place anyone in danger and therefore require special precautions.

9. Consider the effect of plant down-time during maintenance. Duty and standby facilities, or some level of redundancy, should be provided where it is essential for system operation to be maintained.

10. Consider providing modular plant to keep the service in operation during maintenance.

11. Consider the likely availability of spares during the plant lifetime, and avoid the use of plant for which spares may be unavailable or in short supply, this may be the case for plant that is about to be superseded.

Installation, operation and control

12. Standard design guidance should be followed regarding the provision of maintenance equipment on all systems, such as drain points, isolating valves and access panels.

13. Consider the water content of pipework and check that there are sufficient drain points so that the system can be drained within a reasonable period.

14. Provide lifting beams above heavy plant items.

15. Check the lift capacity if there is a likelihood that these will be used to transport plant to roof plant rooms, including replacement plant.

16. Check that all plant and systems can be monitored and connected to a building management system, if applicable.

Access

17. Check the occupancy patterns to determine when access for maintenance will be possible.

18. Inform architects and other design team members of the access requirements for maintenance. Access panels in ceilings, particularly in toilets, are typical areas of potential conflict.

19. Check there is adequate access in and around the site for installation, maintenance and deliveries for all services. Inform other design team members of requirements at an early stage, including those to facilitate replacement of major plant during the building life.

20. The layout of plant systems should permit adequate access for maintenance; check manufacturers' guidelines.

21. Allow sufficient space for access for commissioning and maintenance.

Economics

22. Designing for maintenance can substantially reduce whole life costs.

6   WHOLE LIFE COSTING

Project title .... **Project No.** .... **Design stage** ....

Engineer .... **Revision No** .... **Date** ....

Checked by .... **Approved by** .... **Date** ....

Design inputs

✓

Notes / Design file cross-reference

- Detail of base case and its alternatives ☐

- Mean time between failure (MTBF) and mean time to repair (MTTR) data (where business impacts of failure are to be included) ☐

- Client assessment of cost of impact of failure ☐

- Utility costs information, including prediction of cost increase ☐

- Client required discount rate ☐

- Other costs ☐

Design outputs

✓

Notes / Design file cross-reference

- Whole-life cost analysis of base case and its alternatives ☐

- Sensitivity analysis ☐

- Agree whole-life cost outputs ☐

Key design checks

✓

Notes / Design file cross-reference

- Are client requirements being met? ☐

- Are all options technically feasible, and do they meet client requirements and legislation? ☐

- Have all relevant costs been included? ☐

- Is the input data current and valid? ☐

- Have all assumptions been agreed with the client? ☐

- Where necessary, does the analysis include data from other disciplines (for example plant room and riser space)? ☐

- Have alteration costs been properly estimated and does the year of occurrence coincide with the client's business plan? ☐

- Has the cost of disposal been correctly estimated to include waste treatment costs where applicable? ☐

- Have health and safety costs and benefits been included in the analysis? ☐

Project specific checks and notes

✓

Notes / Design file cross-reference

☐

☐

6 WHOLE LIFE COSTING

Design inputs

- Detail of base case and its alternatives:
  - Capital costs (including temporary works)
  - Tax allowances where applicable
  - Installation costs (including temporary works)
  - Operational costs (including hours of operation, facility and staff costs)
  - Maintenance costs (routine/in-house/outsourced/special – including facility, business, business disruption and staff costs)
  - De-commissioning and disposal costs (equipment/facility/business/temporary works)
  - Energy usage data
  - Water consumption data
  - Equipment life data (and under what conditions this value provided)
  - Equipment footprint and work space requirements.
- Expected lives for components and equipment agreed with client
- Expected maintenance activities and frequency agreed with client in the context of their maintenance strategy or policies and experience (manufacturers may have useful information)
- Period of analysis in years
- Mean time between failure (MTBF) and mean time to repair (MTTR) data (where business impacts of failure are to be included)
- Client assessment of cost of impact of failure
- Utility costs information, including prediction of cost increase
- Client required discount rate

See also: Maintenance, Design Margins, Future Needs

- Other costs:
  - Central support services
  - Administration
  - Overheads
  - Consultancy fees
  - Expenses (financial, technical and legal)
  - Land costs where appropriate
  - Wayleave and compensation costs where appropriate
  - Insurance costs
  - Materials recycling (pipework)
  - Environmental consequences of materials' production and disposal.

Design outputs

- Whole-life cost analysis of base case and its alternatives
- Sensitivity analysis
- Agree whole-life cost outputs

Key design checks

- Are client requirements being met?
- Are all options technically feasible, do they meet client requirements and legislation?
- Have all relevant costs been included?
- Is the input data current and valid?
- Have all assumptions been agreed with the client?
- Where necessary, does the analysis include data from other disciplines (for example plant room and riser space)?
- Have alteration costs been properly estimated and does the year of occurrence coincide with the client's business plan?
- Has the cost of disposal been correctly estimated to include waste treatment costs where applicable?
- Have health and safety costs and benefits been included in the analysis?

DESIGN WATCHPOINTS

Design watchpoints

1. Is the range of alternatives being considered wide enough or are minor variants of one theme being considered?
2. Has any potentially lower whole life cost alternative been ruled out due to technical feasibility or other constraints (legal, political and financial)?
3. Can overall options be split into independent components where separable components may provide better value than others?
4. Has account been taken of:
   - Operating costs including contingency costs and residual value, staff costs including overhead, maintenance and administration
   - Other costs and benefits which may be valued in money terms (such as business efficiencies, deficiencies and disruption costs)
   - Description of those costs and benefits which cannot be easily valued in financial terms?
5. Have all costs and benefits been expressed in real terms and discounted at the appropriate rate?
6. Have costs been estimated properly?
7. Have adjustments been made for taxes and subsidies where appropriate?

8. Have all important risks and uncertainties been identified for the base case and each alternative?
9. Is the costing period long enough to encompass all-important costs and benefits?
10. Are costs estimated from generic data (such as floor area cost per square metre)? If so, what level of accuracy is expected?
11. Consider whole life cost options in a broader context of building design and overall building services strategy.
12. Take account of opportunities for material recycling.
13. Check that disposal costs are included where applicable.
14. When agreeing whole life cost outputs, consider that typical measures include a rate per component or functional unit per year at net present values, or ratio of through-life costs at net present values to capital costs for x years.
15. Guidance on economic service lives of components is provided in the *CIBSE Publication Guide to Ownership, Operation and Maintenance of Building Services.*
16. Guidance on expected component service lives, maintenance activities and frequencies, modes and causes of failure can be obtained from the BLP Construction Durability Database – www.componentlife.com.

7   HEALTH AND SAFETY

Project title.. **Project No.**.. **Design stage**..................

Engineer... **Revision No**... **Date**.............................

Checked by.. **Approved by**...................................... **Date**.............................

Design inputs

✓ **Notes / Design file cross-reference**

- Minimum space requirements for:
  - Installation
  - Commissioning
  - Operation
  - Maintenance
  - De-commissioning ❑

- Environmental conditions required by equipment ❑

- Details of proposed system design ❑

Design outputs

✓ **Notes / Design file cross-reference**

- Risk analysis and management documentation ❑

- Health and safety plan ❑

- Health and safety file ❑

- Risk management documentation ❑

- Revised design details ❑

Key design checks

✓ **Notes / Design file cross-reference**

- Check for compliance with relevant regulations and associated approved codes of practice ❑

Project specific checks and notes

✓ **Notes / Design file cross-reference**

❑

❑

❑

© BSRIA BG2/2006

7   HEALTH AND SAFETY

Why consider this?

- Legislative requirement
  - Installation
  - Commissioning
  - Maintenance
  - De-commissioning
  - Reduced OandM costs

Design inputs

- Minimum space requirements for:
  - Installation
  - Commissioning
  - Operation
  - Maintenance
  - De-commissioning
- Environmental conditions required by equipment
- Details of proposed system design

Design outputs

- Risk analysis and management documentation
- Health and safety plan
- Health and safety file
- Risk management documentation
- Revised design details

Key design checks

- Check for compliance with relevant regulations and associated approved codes of practice

DESIGN WATCHPOINTS

General watchpoints

1. Check for compliance with the *Construction (Design and Management) Regulations*. The following are relevant:
   - Check that clients will be made aware of their duties
   - Provide adequate information concerning health and safety risk issues relating to the design to relevant parties
   - Co-operate with the planning supervisor and, where appropriate, other designers involved in the project
   - Identify the significant health and safety hazards associated with the design and their impact on the construction and operation/maintenance phases
   - Consider the risk from hazards that will arise as a result of the design Consider how this risk can be reduced or avoided
   - Check that information will be provided concerning risks that cannot be designed out
   - Check that relevant information will be provided to the planning supervisor and other designers.

2. Check for compliance with the *Control of Substances Hazardous to Health Regulations (COSHH)*.

3. Check whether the system design could result in the use of hazardous substances. Where possible design out the use of hazardous substances.

4. Where the use of hazardous substances cannot be designed out, check what design considerations could result in the number of personnel exposed to the substances reduced to a minimum, along with the level and duration of exposure.

5. Check for compliance with the *Confined Spaces Regulations*.

6. Check that the necessity for personnel to enter confined spaces has been designed out where possible.

7. Check that plant/equipment associated with confined spaces can be isolated.

8. Check that entrances to confined spaces will be large enough to allow personnel to easily exit the space. Consider the extra space requirement associated with the wearing of protective clothing.

9. Check the ventilation requirements of confined spaces.

10. Check for compliance with the *Work at Height Regulations*.

11. Check whether the design minimises, as far as is practical, the requirement for working at height.

12. Where working at height cannot be designed out check that appropriate protective measures are specified, such as guard rails.

13. Check that the design and installation of the system/equipment will meet the requirements of the *Provision and Use of Work Equipment Regulations*.

14. Allow sufficient space/access for safe working on equipment.

15. Check that the requirements of *HSC L8 – The Control of Legionella Bacteria in Water Systems* have been met. Check that the guidance provided in *Legionnaires' Disease – Cold Water Services* and *Legionnaires' Disease – Hot Water Services* has been considered.

16. Check that the requirements of the *Water Supply (Water Fittings) Regulations* and associated *Water Regulations Guide* are met.

17. Check that the requirements of *Safe Working in Sewers and at Sewage Works* published by The Joint Health and Safety Committee for the Water Service are met.

8   SITE LOCATION FACTORS

Project title.. **Project No.**.. **Design stage**...................

Engineer... **Revision No**...................................... **Date**..............................

Checked by.. **Approved by**...................................... **Date**..............................

Design inputs

- Precise site location details ☐
- Details of surrounding buildings and infrastructure ☐
- Details of planned site development, including planned shape and form ☐
- Positions and details of existing utilities and their capabilities ☐
- Details of water supply availability, reliability and quality ☐
- Details of previous site occupancy, possible hazardous wastes, such as contaminated land and gases ☐
- Details of foul and surface water sewers for their location, capacity and level ☐
- Ownership of sewers such as private or water authority ☐

Notes / Design file cross-reference

Design outputs

- Site assessment covering local infrastructure and pollution ☐
- Site survey report with details of soil conditions and buried services ☐

Notes / Design file cross-reference

Key design checks

- Check if any sub-terrain tunnels or services run through the site ☐
- Check whether the incoming water supply main has sufficient capacity and pressure for the site requirements, including required temporary supply and system flushing requirements ☐
- Check and agree utility and local authority requirements ☐
- Check the water disposal requirements of the Environment Agency and local water authority ☐
- Check planning requirements ☐
- Check to confirm no services require diversion or relocation ☐
- Check distance is at least 3·0 m from adopted sewers ☐

Notes / Design file cross-reference

8   SITE LOCATION FACTORS

Project title.. **Project No**... **Design stage**......................

Engineer.. **Revision No**... **Date**......................................

Checked by... **Approved by** .... **Date**....................................

Key design checks (cont.)

✓ **Notes / Design file cross-reference**

- Check existing wayleaves ☐

- Check existing rights to drainage (ownership) ☐

- Check flood risk, for example whether the site is in a flood plain ☐

- Check existing drainage levels ☐

- Check storm design criteria with the Environment Agency ☐

- On site surface-water storage requirements ☐

- Check that the drainage can be achieved by gravity ☐

Project specific checks and notes

✓ **Notes / Design file cross-reference**

☐

☐

☐

© BSRIA BG2/2006

8 SITE LOCATION FACTORS

Design inputs

- Precise site location details
- Details of surrounding buildings and infrastructure
- Details of planned site development, including planned shape and form
- Positions and details of existing utilities and their capabilities
- Details of water supply availability, reliability and quality
- Details of previous site occupancy, possible hazardous wastes, such as contaminated land and gases
- Details of foul and surface water sewers with the location, capacity and level
- Ownership of sewers such as private or water authority

Design information

- Local authority and other statutory requirements such as environmental health, and the specific requirements of the NRA, Environment Agency, planning, building control, fire officer, water authorities and utility companies
- Details of site water table
- Details of buried services involving a comprehensive survey including ground penetration radar where appropriate

See also: Local Authority Requirements and Discharge Consents

Design outputs

- Site assessment covering local infrastructure and pollution
- Site survey report with details of soil conditions and buried services

Key design checks

- Check if any sub-terrain tunnels or services run through the site
- Check whether the incoming water supply main has sufficient capacity and pressure for site requirements, including required temporary supply and system flushing requirements
- Check and agree utility and local authority requirements
- Check the water disposal requirements of the Environment Agency and local water authority
- Check planning requirements
- Check to confirm no services require diversion or relocation
- Check distance is at least 3·0 m from adopted sewers
- Check existing wayleaves
- Check existing rights to drainage (ownership)
- Check flood risk, for example whether the site is in a flood plain
- Check existing drainage levels
- Check storm design criteria with the Environment Agency
- On site surface-water storage requirements
- Check that the drainage can be achieved by gravity

DESIGN WATCHPOINTS

General watchpoints

1. Check on sewer surcharge levels.
2. Prevent flooding of basements by pumping over.
3. Agree specific site and design data with client as necessary.
4. Site visits, where possible, can provide useful data for design and should be properly documented with photographs of surroundings.
5. Where site visits are not possible, such as for overseas locations, full information on location must be obtained via the client or client's representative.
6. Check local water supply quality and hardness with the relevant water board to assess treatment requirements. It may be necessary to test a sample of mains water.

7. The effects of increased corrosion risk must be considered for coastal locations.
8. Check if any sub-terrain tunnels or services run through site such as sewerage, tubes or transportation systems.
9. Check that all relevant drawings are received from utility companies and check location of services and connection points. Surveys may be required. Check ease of access for testing condition and location.
10. Check and agree utility and local authority requirements.
11. Check access to site, for construction access, deliveries, and for future plant and equipment replacement requirements.
12. Check maximum boundary noise levels from plant and equipment.

9 LOCAL AUTHORITY REQUIREMENTS AND DISCHARGE CONSENTS

Project title.. **Project No**.. **Design stage**....................

Engineer... **Revision No** .... **Date** ....

Checked by.. **Approved by** .... **Date** ....

Design inputs

✓ **Notes / Design file cross-reference**

- Number and location of all sanitary appliances and other equipment which may discharge to drain ❏

- If relevant, obtain the location, size, invert levels and direction of flow of all existing foul and surface water sewers ❏

- Determine whether foul and surface water sewers are combined or separate systems ❏

- Determine whether existing systems are private or public sewers ❏

- Requirement for a Building Over Agreement (permission required from sewerage undertaker to build over the top of or within 3 m of a public sewer) ❏

- Any recorded sewer surcharge levels ❏

- Level of local water table ❏

Design outputs

✓ **Notes / Design file cross-reference**

- Determine maximum flow rate for both foul and surface water drainage ❏

- Check whether foul or surface water retention is required (including sustainable urban drainage requirements) ❏

- Check whether the systems are to be separate or combined ❏

- Provide the drainage authority with all information necessary for it to issue a Discharge Consent, if applicable ❏

- If new sewers are to be installed check whether they are to be adopted by the sewerage provider ❏

- Possible use of sewage treatment on-site, such as reed beds ❏

Key design checks

✓ **Notes / Design file cross-reference**

- Design in accordance with *Approved Document H – Drainage and Waste Disposal* ❏

- Design in accordance with *BS EN 12056 – Gravity drainage system inside buildings BS EN 752 Drain and sewer systems outside buildings and BS EN 1610 - Construction and testing of drains and sewers* ❏

© BSRIA BG2/2006

9   LOCAL AUTHORITY REQUIREMENTS AND DISCHARGE CONSENTS

Project title.. **Project No**.. **Design stage**.....................

Engineer.. **Revision No** .... **Date**.......................................

Checked by... **Approved by** .... **Date**.......................................

Key design checks (cont.)

- If applicable, check that the necessary Discharge Consent is required from the Environment Agency in order to discharge into controlled waters, in accordance with the *Water Resources Act 1991*. Check the quality of discharge required

- If applicable, check that the necessary Discharge Consent is required from the sewerage provider in order to discharge into a sewer in accordance with the *Water Industry Act 1991*

- Check that no trade wastes will be discharged

- Check for compliance with Environment Agency's *PPG3*

Notes / Design file cross-reference

Project specific checks and notes

Notes / Design file cross-reference

© BSRIA BG2/2006

9 LOCAL AUTHORITY REQUIREMENTS AND DISCHARGE CONSENTS

Design inputs

- Number and location of all sanitary appliances and other equipment which may discharge to drain
- If relevant, obtain the location, size, invert levels and direction of flow of all existing foul and surface water sewers
- Determine whether foul and surface water sewers are combined or separate systems
- Determine whether existing systems are private or public sewers
- Requirement for a Building Over Agreement (permission required from sewerage undertaker to build over the top of or within 3 m of a public sewer)
- Any recorded sewer surcharge levels
- Level of local water table

Design information

- Building type and use
- Occupancy patterns
- Check whether existing sewers are available
- Limitations on the rate of discharge into any private or public sewers, or into any controlled waters as stipulated by the sewerage provider
- Check whether the existing sewers are private or public
- Check the presence of trade waste

Design outputs

- Determine the maximum flow rate for both foul and surface water drainage
- Check whether foul or surface water retention is required (including sustainable urban drainage requirements)
- Check whether the systems are to be separate or combined

- Provide the drainage authority with all information necessary for it to issue a Discharge Consent if applicable
- If new sewers are to be installed check whether they are to be adopted by the sewerage provider
- Check the possible use of on-site sewage treatment, such as reed beds

Key design checks

- Design in accordance with *Approved Document H – Drainage and Waste Disposal*
- Design in accordance with *BS EN 12056 – Gravity drainage systems inside buildings BS EN 752 Drain and sewer systems outside buildings* and *BS EN 1610 - Construction and testing of drains and sewers*
- If applicable, check that the necessary Discharge Consent is required from the Environment Agency in order to discharge into controlled waters (surface water) in accordance with the *Water Resources Act 1991*. Check quality of discharge required
- If applicable, check that the necessary Discharge Consent is required from the sewerage provider (foul water) in order to discharge into a sewer in accordance with the *Water Industry Act 1991*
- Check that no trade wastes will be discharged
- Check for compliance with Environment Agency's *PPG3*

See also: Foul Water Below Ground Drainage Systems, Commercial Kitchen Drainage, Surface Water Below Ground Drainage Systems, Roof Drainage, Sustainable Urban Drainage Systems

---

DESIGN WATCHPOINTS

Sizing and selection

1. Check that the drainage system is designed and installed so that there is adequate hydraulic capacity.
2. Follow requirements of the planning consent.
3. Check that the drainage system is water and gas tight against operational pressures. Check that vapours and foul air will not be released into the building.
4. Check that provision is made to avoid flooding into the building if there is a risk of flooding from the external drainage system. Follow the requirements of BS EN 12056-4.
5. Check that no poisonous, noxious or polluting material is discharged into any controlled waters, either deliberately or accidentally, without a consent for that discharge.
6. If discharging into a private or public sewer or controlled waters, check that the maximum flow rate, as stipulated by the sewerage provider or Environment Agency, has not been exceeded. Consider the use of a vortex device to restrict the flow to a predetermined maximum. Check that the drainage is not to ground in the ground water protection zone.
7. Check that adequate provision has been provided when discharging into controlled waters so that the banks and bed of the watercourse are not eroded due to the incoming flow.
8. Check that if a new sewer is to be adopted by the sewerage provider, that it is designed in accordance with the latest edition of *Sewers for Adoption*.

9. Check that any surface water which may have become polluted with oils or fuel passes through a petrol interceptor before discharging into any sewer or controlled waters. Environment Agency *PPG3*.
10. Check that the maximum stipulated flow rate has not been exceeded when discharging from underground storage via automatic wastewater lifting plant. Follow the requirements in *BS EN 752 – 6*.
11. Consider the use of on-site treatment plant if sewers are not available.
12. Consider special requirements for fuel-filling stations.

Installation, operation and control

13. Consider marking separate systems of drainage as recommended by the Environment Agency, such as red for foul drains and blue for surface water drains.
14. Note that sites with interceptors must be registered under the *Hazardous Waste Regulations*.

Economics

15. The sewerage provider and the Environment Agency will generally make a charge for issuing the discharge consent.
16. An estimate or a quotation will be given by the sewerage provider or the EA once all the relevant design information has been supplied by the client or the representative.
17. Under normal circumstances these charges will be paid prior to any consent being issued.

10 MAINS WATER AVAILABILITY

Project title .... **Project No.** .... **Design stage** ....

Engineer .... **Revision No** .... **Date** ....

Checked by .... **Approved by** .... **Date** ....

Design inputs

✓ **Notes / Design file cross-reference**

- Details of the application, such as the type of building and its function, number of occupants and sanitary appliances and whether these are permanent or transitional ☐

- Period and hours of occupation and pattern of water use ☐

- Details of available water quantities and pressures during peak conditions from the water supply company ☐

- Possible location of incoming supply and internal supplies ☐

- Check whether a bore hole supply is a viable option, if required ☐

- Quantity of on-site cold water storage (if any) ☐

- Required mains-water flow rate and pressure and allowance for possible future reduction in pressure ☐

Design outputs

✓ **Notes / Design file cross-reference**

- Size and location of internal mains water services ☐

- Requirements for dual supplies from separate mains ☐

- Requirement for backflow prevention devices – categories of protection in accordance with the *Water Regulations* ☐

- Requirement for fire protection services such as sprinklers and hose reels ☐

- Provide the water undertaker with all information necessary for it to determine the size of service pipe to be installed ☐

- Requirement for water storage and booster pumps ☐

© BSRIA BG2/2006

10   MAINS WATER AVAILABILITY

Project title ....   **Project No.** ....   **Design stage** ....

Engineer ....   **Revision No** ....   **Date** ....

Checked by ....   **Approved by** ....   **Date** ....

Key design checks

✓   **Notes / Design file cross-reference**

- Systems have to comply with the *Water Supply (Water Fittings) Regulations 1999* and the *Water Byelaws 2000, Scotland* and the associated *Water Regulations Guide*

  ☐

- Systems should be designed in accordance with *BS 6700 and BS EN 806-2*

  ☐

- Compliance with *Health and Safety Commission ACOP L8*

  ☐

Project specific checks and notes

✓   **Notes / Design file cross-reference**

☐

☐

☐

© BSRIA BG2/2006

10 MAINS WATER AVAILABILITY

Design inputs

- Details of the application, such as the type of building and its function, number of occupants and sanitary appliances and whether they are permanent or transitional
- Period and hours of occupation and pattern of water use
- Details of available water quantities and pressures during peak conditions from the water supply company
- Possible location of incoming supply and internal supplies
- Check whether a bore hole supply is a viable option, if required
- Quantity of on-site cold water storage (if any)
- Required mains-water flow rate and pressure and allowance for possible future reduction in pressure

Design information

- Obtain the location, size and pressure of water supply in the locality of the building or site from the water undertaker
- Chemical and biological constituents of water supply - mains or borehole

See also: Contamination Prevention, Pipe Sizing – Cold and Hot Water Services, Cold Water Storage and Distribution, Legionnaires' Disease– Cold Water Services, Pressure Boosting of Water, Fire Systems – Water Supply.

Design outputs

- Size and location of internal mains water services
- Requirements for dual supplies from separate mains
- Requirement for backflow prevention devices – categories of protection in accordance with the *Water Regulations*
- Requirement for fire protection services such as sprinklers and hose reels
- Provide the water undertaker with all information necessary for it to determine the size of service pipe to be installed
- Requirement for water storage and booster pumps

Key design checks

- Systems have to comply with the *Water Supply (Water Fittings) Regulations 1999*, the *Water Byelaws 2000, Scotland* and the associated *Water Regulations Guide*
- Systems should be designed in accordance with *BS 6700 and BS EN 806-2*
- Compliance with *Health and Safety Commission ACOP L8*

DESIGN WATCHPOINTS

Sizing and selection

1. Consider whether all fittings shall be supplied directly from mains water supply.
2. Determine the hardness of the incoming water supply and consider water treatment if necessary such as softening and conditioning.
3. Check that there are no cross connections between the water undertaker's supply and any water from another source, such as a borehole.
4. Determine what lead-in time the water undertaker requires for the installation of the service pipe, and whether this is in accordance with the construction programme.
5. Check that provision has been allowed for the installation of a water meter.
6. If insufficient pressure is available or cannot be maintained, then consideration must be given to the installation of a boosted water system. (See Pressure Boosting of Water)
7. Consider the risk of frost damage. The location of pipes, cisterns and system components must be considered. If frost damage is possible, protection should be provided in accordance with BS 6700 and the *Water Regulations Guide*.
8. Check services are colour banded in accordance with BS 1710:1984.
9. Consider sterilisation of the system in accordance with BS 6700:1997.

Installation, operation and control

10. Check that all pipework, appliances and controls do not obstruct users.
11. Check that pipework and fixings are enclosed to deter vandalism and avoid accidental damage.
12. Check that the incoming service pipe can be installed at the minimum depth of 750 mm.

Access and maintenance

13. Check that the stop valve on the boundary is in an accessible position.

Economics

14. The water undertaker will generally make a charge for the installation of the service pipe and any necessary infrastructure works.
15. An estimate or quotation will be given by the water undertaker once all the relevant design information has been supplied by the client or its representative.
16. Under normal circumstances charges will be paid prior to any water connection being made.

11 CONTAMINATION PREVENTION

Project title .... **Project No**. .... **Design stage** ....

Engineer .... **Revision No** .... **Date** ....

Checked by .... **Approved by** .... **Date** ....

Design inputs

- Design flow rates and pressures required in the system

□ **Notes / Design file cross-reference**

Design outputs

- Type of backflow prevention arrangements and devices required

□

- Required location and installation requirements for backflow prevention arrangements and devices

□ **Notes / Design file cross-reference**

Key design checks

- Check that the requirements of the *Water Supply (Water Fittings) Regulations 1999*, the *Water Byelaws 2000 Scotland* and the associated *Water Regulations Guide* are met

□ **Notes / Design file cross-reference**

- Check that appropriate backflow prevention arrangements and devices are selected in relation to the fluid category, appliance and system design (See *Water Regulations Guide*)

□

- Check that water delivered will not be liable to become contaminated

□

- Check that contamination of the water undertaker's supply does not occur

□

Project specific checks and notes

□ **Notes / Design file cross-reference**

□

□

© BSRIA BG2/2006

11 CONTAMINATION PREVENTION

Design inputs

- Design flow rates and pressures required in the system

Design information

- Type of appliances to be included in the system both mechanical and non-mechanical
- Fluid categories that will be present in the system

Design outputs

- Type of backflow prevention arrangements and devices required
- Required location and installation requirements for backflow prevention arrangements and devices

See also: Cold Water Storage and Distribution, Legionnaires' Disease– Cold Water Services, Legionnaires' Disease – Hot Water Services

Key design checks

- Check that the requirements of the *Water Supply (Water Fittings) Regulations 1999,* the *Water Byelaws 2000 Scotland* and the associated *Water Regulations Guide* are met
- Check that appropriate backflow prevention arrangements and devices are selected in relation to the fluid category, appliance and system design (See the *Water Regulations Guide*)
- Check that water delivered will not be liable to become contaminated
- Check that contamination of the water undertaker's supply does not occur

DESIGN WATCHPOINTS

Sizing and selection

1. Check that all backflow prevention devices are approved by Water Regulations Advisory Scheme (WRAS).
2. Check that the correct water fluid category (1 to 5) has been identified. Fluid categories range from 1 (wholesome water) to 5 (water representing a serious health hazard).
3. Check that backflow prevention arrangements and devices will be appropriate for the highest applicable fluid category.
4. Check that backflow protection will be provided on any supply pipe where it is necessary to prevent backflow between separate premises.
5. Check that materials to be in contact with the water will be suitable for the purpose.
6. Check that no pump will be connected directly to the water undertaker's supply without its prior written approval. (The *Water Regulations* limit pump sizes to 12 l/min maximum for direct connection to mains water.)

Installation, operation and control

7. Check that no cross-connection will occur between pipes conveying water supplied by the water undertaker with pipes conveying water from another supplier.
8. Check that stagnation, particularly at high temperatures, will not occur.
9. Check that pipes and cisterns containing non-wholesome water will be marked or colour coded in accordance with BS 1710.
10. Check that colour identification will be placed at all junctions, inlets/outlets of valves and appliances, and where pipes pass through walls at points adjacent to both wall surfaces.
11. Check that an appropriate backflow prevention device is installed where a pipe carrying non-wholesome water is to be connected to one carrying wholesome water.

12. Check that an appropriate backflow prevention arrangement or device is fitted for any appliance, fitting or process. This is with the exception of water heaters that allow expanded water to flow back into the supply pipe; vented water storage vessels (supplied from a storage system) or where the water temperature in the cistern or supply pipe does not exceed 25°C.
13. Check that adequate air gaps will be provided where required, such as for cisterns, basins and baths.
14. Check that backflow prevention devices are not normally located outside premises – with the exception of types *HA* and *HUK1* for protection against fluid categories 2 and 3.
15. Check that vented or verifiable devices, or devices with relief outlets will not be installed in chambers below ground level or where flooding is possible.
16. Check that backflow prevention devices, such as an RPZ valve (see table), for fluid category 4 will be provided with line strainers immediately upstream. Check that servicing valves will be fitted upstream of line strainers and immediately downstream of the backflow prevention device.
17. Check that, where a reduced pressure zone valve is to be fitted, the relief outlet will terminate with a Type AA air gap located a minimum of 300 mm above the ground or floor level.
18. Check that the requirements in table 1 for backflow prevention devices are met.

Access and maintenance

19. Check that backflow devices will be accessible for inspection, testing, maintenance and renewal.
20. Check that backflow prevention devices will not be buried in the ground.

Table 1: Requirement for backflow prevention.

Type	Backflow prevention device	Requirement
BA	Verifiable backflow preventer with reduced pressure zone (RPZ)	Check that a Type AA air gap will be provided between the relief outlet port and the top of the tundish.
CA	Non-verifiable disconnector with different pressure zones	Check that a Type AA air gap will be provided between the relief outlet port and the top of the tundish.
DA	Anti-vacuum valve	Check that the device will be fitted on a Type A upstand with the outlet not less than 300 mm above the discharge point or spill-over level. Check that no valve, flow restrictor, or tap will be fitted on the outlet of the device.
DB	Pipe interrupter with vent and moving element	Check that the device will be fitted with the lowest point of the air aperture not less than 300 mm above the discharge point or spill-over level. Check that no valve, flow restrictor, or tap will be fitted on the outlet of the device.
DC	Pipe interrupter with permanent atmospheric vent	With the exception of urinals, check that the device will be fitted with the lowest point of the air aperture not less than 300 mm above the discharge point or spill-over level. Check that no valve, flow restrictor, or tap will be fitted on the outlet of the device. For urinals check that the device will be fitted not less than 150 mm above the sparge outlet.
DUK1	Anti-vacuum valve combined with verifiable check valve	Check that the device will be fitted on a Type B upstand with the outlet not less than 300 mm above the discharge point or spill-over level. Check that no valve, flow restrictor, or tap will be fitted on the outlet of the device.
LA	Pressure air inlet valve	Check that use will be limited to locations where operational waste is acceptable, such as gardens or similar.
LB	Pressurised air inlet valve combined with check valve downstream	Check that use will be limited to locations where operational waste is acceptable, such as gardens or similar.

12   WATER CONSERVATION

Project title... **Project No**................................... **Design stage**....................

Engineer... **Revision No**................................. **Date**..

Checked by.. **Approved by**................................... **Date**................................

Design inputs

- Number of occupants

- Non-domestic use

- Occupancy patterns

✓ **Notes / Design file cross-reference**

❑

❑

❑

Design outputs

- Suitable methods to conserve water

- Appropriate backflow prevention

✓ **Notes / Design file cross-reference**

❑

❑

Key design checks

- Check that the design and associated components comply with the *Water Supply (Water Fittings) Regulations 1999*, the *Water Byelaws 2000 Scotland* and the associated *Water Regulations Guide*

- Check that the design and associated components comply with *BS 6700* and *BS EN 806-2*

✓ **Notes / Design file cross-reference**

❑

❑

Project specific checks and notes

✓ **Notes / Design file cross-reference**

❑

❑

❑

12 WATER CONSERVATION

Design inputs

- Number of occupants
- Non–domestic use
- Occupancy patterns

Design information

- Building use, type and occupational patterns
- Supply water quality
- Type of sanitary fittings and other sources of water consumption

See also: Contamination Prevention, Cold Water Distribution and Storage, Hot Water Storage and Distribution, Reclaimed Water Systems – Greywater, Reclaimed Water Systems – Rainwater

Design outputs

- Suitable methods to conserve water
- Appropriate backflow prevention

Key design checks

- Check that the design and associated components comply with the *Water Supply (Water Fittings) Regulations 1999*, the *Water Byelaws 2000 Scotland*, and the associated *Water Regulations Guide*
- Check that the design and associated components comply with *BS 6700* and *BS EN 806-2*

DESIGN WATCHPOINTS

Sizing and selection

1. Check that the selected water closet pans (WC) satisfy the flushing requirements of *BS EN 997:2003*.
2. Check that flushing volumes for WC cisterns will not exceed six litres. Check that dual-flush cisterns provide a maximum flush of six and four litres respectively.
3. Check that a cistern serving a single urinal will be filled with water at a rate not exceeding 10 l/h.
4. Check that cisterns serving two or more urinal bowls or urinal slab positions will be filled with water at a rate not exceeding 7·5 l/h per bowl or 700 mm length of slab. Select an appropriate means of controlling the water supply: time control, passive infrared (PIR) control, or hydraulic control. For the former, check that a lockable control valve will be fitted. (Note that 10 l/h and 7 l/h requirements do not apply where PIR controls are fitted.)
5. For lightly used urinals, consider the use of a user-actuated flush for individual bowls and stalls. Check that the flush will not exceed 1·5 litres. Consider the use of manual chain pulls, push buttons or occupancy sensors, such as an infra-red sensor.
6. Check that appropriate backflow prevention devices (pipe interceptor with permanent atmospheric vent) are selected for pressure flushing cisterns and pressure flushing valves for WCs and urinals.
7. Check that self-closing taps will be of the non-concussive type and capable of closing against two and a half times the working pressure without leakage. This should also be the case for radar and PIR operated taps and valves, and electronic WC flushing.
8. Consider the use of low-flow showers and flow restrictors.
9. Consider the use of spray taps or aerators. Spray taps are not appropriate where there may be heavy fouling of basins by grease and dirt. In hard water areas, a blockage of the spray head may occur. In soft water areas a build-up of grease and soap residue in waste pipes can occur.
10. Check that in-line filters will be installed for flow restrictors and aerators to prevent blockage by water-borne particles.
11. Consider use of electronic controls using PIRs to isolate water supply in toilets.
12. Consider the use of proximity sensor operated taps.
13. Consider the use of automatic leak detection devices.
14. Consider the use of waterless urinals.

Installation, operation and control

15. Check that warning pipes from cisterns and discharge pipes from relief valves will be located so that any flow of water is apparent.
16. Check that adequate frost precautions will be taken.
17. Check that approved fittings, components and pipes will be used.
18. Check that protection from mechanical damage and corrosion will be provided (especially underground). Check for proper trench preparation, backfill and pipe depth.

Access and maintenance

19. Consider that self-closing taps should only be used where regular inspection and maintenance can be ensured.
20. Spray taps and aerators will require regular maintenance.
21. Check that filters, aerators and terminal flow restrictors will be easily removable for cleaning.
22. Be aware that waterless urinals will require regular maintenance.
23. Be aware that WC pans fitted with cisterns that have internal overflows require regular inspection to witness overflow water running into the WC pan.

Economics

24. Consider selecting equipment listed on the water technology product list for enhanced capital allowances.
25. Where necessary, check that adequate provision will be provided to monitor the water usage/discharge via the building management system.
26. Consider whole-life costs of suitable options.

CALCULATIONS

13   COMPUTER CALCULATIONS

Project title.. **Project No**... **Design stage**...................

Engineer.. **Revision No**...................................... **Date**.................................

Checked by.. **Approved by**.................................. **Date**.................................

Design inputs
☑ **Notes / Design file cross-reference**

- Design data relevant to the computer design package being used ☐

Design outputs
☑ **Notes / Design file cross-reference**

- Printout or other record of all actual as-entered inputs to the package, clearly cross-referenced to the design file ☐

- Hardcopy of all output, clearly cross-referenced to the design file ☐

Key design checks
☑ **Notes / Design file cross-reference**

- Check that any software package has been validated and is suitable for the intended application ☐

- Record any assumptions made because input information is not available, and mark to redo and check when information is received ☐

- Check the assumptions introduced into the software calculations ☐

- Record all actual inputs to the design software, by printout or screen dump ☐

- Cross-check all outputs against reasonable benchmarks ☐

- Review any margins added at any of the calculation stages; these should be justified (and recorded in the design file) or removed ☐

Project specific checks and notes
☑ **Notes / Design file cross-reference**

☐
☐
☐

© BSRIA BG2/2006

13 COMPUTER CALCULATIONS

Design inputs

- Design data relevant to the computer design package being used

Design outputs

- Printout or other record of all actual as-entered inputs to the package, clearly cross-referenced to the design file
- Hardcopy of all output, clearly cross-referenced to the design file

See also: Design Margins, Future Needs, All calculation sheets

Key design checks

- Check that any software package has been validated and is suitable for the intended application
- Record any assumptions made because input information is not available, and mark to redo and check when information is received
- Check any assumptions made by the program
- Record all actual inputs to the design package, by printout or screen dump
- Cross check all outputs against reasonable benchmarks
- Review any margins added at any of the calculation stages; these should be justified (and recorded in the design file) or removed

DESIGN WATCHPOINTS

General watchpoints

1. Check that any software package has been validated and is suitable for the intended application, in other words whether it will carry out the required tasks to an acceptable standard.

2. Avoid the use of other engineer's spreadsheets as they may not have gone through a quality assurance procedure of verification and validation.

3. Check and record the basis used for the calculation. Basic evaluation of software should always be carried out to check the design basis. This should also be done for each revision of current software packages.

4. Record and check all actual inputs to the design package, by printout or screen dump. Never assume that input data has been entered correctly – always check.

5. Check all results and the output for any obvious errors. Cross check all outputs against reasonable benchmarks or rules of thumb.

6. Check any assumptions made by the program.

7. Record any assumptions made when input information is not available and mark to redo and check when information is received.

8. Review any margins added at any of the calculation stages, and check whether these are justified. Reasons for use should be recorded in the design file. If used because required input data is not available, record and revisit when the data is available.

9. Room dimensions should be as accurate as possible. If using architects' drawings, use the dimensions shown on the drawings wherever possible rather than scaling, as the drawing can become distorted when copied. Check dimensions with the originator if in doubt.

10. Keep an accurate log of any changes during the design process.

Economics

11. Use of computer packages can save time and money, but they are only one of several design tools. It is still the responsibility of the engineer to check the package itself and the inputs and outputs.

14   PIPE SIZING – COLD AND HOT WATER SERVICES

Project title.. **Project No**.. **Design stage**..................

Engineer... **Revision No**.. **Date**................................

Checked by.. **Approved by**...................................... **Date**................................

Design inputs

☑

Notes / Design file cross-reference

- Number and type of appliances   ☐

- Location of appliances   ☐

- Available pressure head (storage cisterns)   ☐

- Minimum mains pressure at time of maximum demand   ☐

Design outputs

☑

Notes / Design file cross-reference

- Size of pipes and associated valves   ☐

- Flow rates and velocities   ☐

- Pipework routes   ☐

- System schematic   ☐

- Requirement for thermal and acoustic insulation   ☐

- Pipework expansion requirements   ☐

- Possible requirement to treat water   ☐

Key design checks

☑

Notes / Design file cross-reference

- Check that the pipe sizing calculations are performed in accordance with *BS 6700* or some other recognised method, such as included in the *Institute of Plumbing Design Guide* or *CIBSE Guide G*   ☐

- Zeta factors for fittings can be obtained from manufacturers' data, or from published tables when specific data is not available   ☐

Project specific checks and notes

☑

Notes / Design file cross-reference

☐

☐

☐

14   PIPE SIZING – COLD AND HOT WATER SERVICES

Design inputs

- Number and type of appliances
- Location of appliances
- Available pressure head (storage cisterns)
- Minimum mains pressure at time of maximum demand

Design information

- Type and use of building
- Pressure-loss characteristics of pipes, valves, taps and other fittings
- Minimum flow rates and pressures for each type of appliance or equipment
- Materials to be used, including copper, plastics, mild steel, stainless steel, and composite materials
- Water quality
- Method of pipework jointing: welded, brazed, soldered, screwed, push-fit, compression and press fit

Design outputs

- Size of pipes and associated valves
- Flow rates and velocities
- Pipework routes
- System schematic
- Requirement for thermal and acoustic insulation
- Pipework expansion requirements
- Possible requirement to treat water

Key design checks

- Check that the pipe sizing calculations are performed in accordance with *BS 6700* or some other recognised method, for example as included in the IOP *Design Guide* or *CIBSE Guide G*
- Zeta factors for fittings can be obtained from manufacturers' data, or from published tables when specific data is not available

See also: Cold Water Storage and Distribution, Hot Water Storage and Distribution, Legionnaires' Disease - Cold Water Services, Legionnaires' Disease Hot - Water Services

DESIGN WATCHPOINTS

Sizing and selection

1. Check that pipework is not sized on the basis of continuous maximum demand (all connected fittings in simultaneous use) unless specifically required to do so by the type of building. Check that the pipework is sized on the basis of probable demand.
2. Check that simultaneous demand is estimated either from data provided by observation and experience of similar installations, or by the use of loading units. (A simultaneous demand calculation method is provided in Annex D of *BS 6700* based on the use of loading units.)
3. Check that loading units are not used to calculate design flow rates in applications were water use is intensive, such as in theatres, conference halls and sports changing room showers. In these instances it is necessary to determine the likely pattern of use and appropriate peak flow demand.
4. Check that constant flow demands, such as urinals, are added to the design flow rate after the loading units have been converted to a flow rate. This should take into consideration the intermittent flow due to the urinal control device.
5. For manual calculations check that the calculation procedure and associated calculation sheet provided in Appendix D of BS 6700 are used.
6. Check that pressure loss or equivalent lengths data are obtained and used for taps, valves and other fittings.
7. Check that appropriate pipe sizing charts are used.
8. For systems supplied from storage cisterns, check that the static head pressure is determined on the basis of the distance from the bottom pipe outlet of the cistern to the point of supply. This will ensure that the system will be designed on the basis of the minimum available pressure.
9. For systems relying on mains pressure, check what the minimum pressure is at the time of peak demand. (This information should be obtained from the water supplier.)
10. Check that maximum velocities in pipework will be low enough to avoid unacceptable noise, such as 3 m/s at 10°C, but high enough to avoid the settling of detritus. (Table 2.19 in *CIBSE Guide G* provides maximum water velocities for different temperatures.). Check that water hammer will be avoided.
11. In high-rise systems, check that outlet fittings on the lower floors are not subjected to excessive pressures (say, above 6 bar). Where necessary consider the use of pressure reducing valves or intermediate level storage systems.
12. Check that no risk of bimetallic corrosion will occur.
13. Consider important issues where pipes are directly associated with the fabric, for example sleeving pipes through walls, the location of notches and holes in beams.

Economics

14. Perform component material specification based on whole-life cost and best value assessment, taking into account durability, time for installation and maintenance requirements and likely refurbishments.
15. Consider minimising different types and sizes of components. The selection of pipe connections, such as soldered, compression fittings, push fittings and press fittings, can have a significant effect on costs.
16. Computer programs can provide a quick and cost effective means of pipe sizing, flow rates, velocities, and probable demand data calculations.

15   PIPE SIZING – ABOVE GROUND SANITARY PIPEWORK

Project title.. **Project No**........................... **Design stage**...............

Engineer... **Revision No**........................... **Date** ....

Checked by .... **Approved by** .... **Date**....................

Design inputs

- Design flow rates from sanitary appliances

- Number of building storeys

- Size of traps associated with sanitary appliances

- Length of discharge branches, intended pipe gradients, number of bends and maximum drop

- Type and nature of building use, number and type of sanitary appliances

Notes / Design file cross-reference

Design outputs

- Size of discharge branches

- Size of discharge stack(s)

- Size of stack ventilation pipe(s)

- Expected maximum design flow rates for sizing underground drainage

Notes / Design file cross-reference

Key design checks

- Check that discharge branches, stacks and vent pipes are calculated in accordance with *Approved Document H1* and/or *BS EN 12056-2*

- Determine the requirement for separate ventilation of branch pipes

- Check that vacuum drainage systems are sized and designed in accordance with *BS EN 12109*

Notes / Design file cross-reference

Project specific checks and notes

Notes / Design file cross-reference

© BSRIA BG2/2006

15 PIPE SIZING – ABOVE GROUND SANITARY PIPEWORK

Design inputs

- Design flow rates from sanitary appliances
- Number of building storeys
- Size of traps associated with sanitary appliances
- Length of discharge branches, intended pipe gradients, number of bends and maximum drop
- Type and nature of building use, number and type of sanitary appliances

Design information

- Location, type and numbers of sanitary appliances
- Vented or un-vented discharge branches
- Specialist discharges are highlighted and/or any continuous flows are known

See also: Sanitary Accommodation Requirements, Drainage Systems-Above Ground Foul Drainage

Design outputs

- Size of discharge branches
- Size of discharge stack(s)
- Size of stack ventilation pipe(s)
- Expected maximum design flow rates for sizing underground drainage

Key design checks

- Check that discharge branches, stacks and vent pipes are calculated in accordance with *Approved Document H1* and/or *BS EN 12056-2*
- Determine the requirement for separate ventilation of branch pipes
- Check that vacuum drainage systems are sized and designed in accordance with *BS EN 12109*

DESIGN WATCHPOINTS

General watchpoints

1. Note that sanitary pipework for domestic and small/ less complex non-domestic buildings should be designed in accordance with *Approved Document H1*. Complex systems in larger buildings should be designed in accordance with *BS EN 12056-2*.

2. Check that the design flowrates are calculated based on discharge units for the preferred sanitary appliances and the appropriate frequency factors. Follow the calculation procedure provided in *BS EN 12056-2*.

3. Sizes and limitations on the use of unvented and ventilated discharge branches are provided in *BS EN 12056-2*. For different pipe diameters this includes: minimum trap seal depth, maximum length of pipe from trap outlet to stack, pipe gradient, maximum number of bends and maximum drop.

4. The hydraulic capacity of both unvented and ventilated discharge branches for a range of nominal pipe diameters is provided in *BS EN 12056-2*.

5. Check that the size and design of branch discharge pipes will not result in occurrence of cross flow.

6. For buildings up to three storeys high, check that discharge branches will be a minimum of 450 mm above the invert level of the rest bend of the drain (in order to prevent back pressure or compression).

7. For buildings up to five storeys high, check that branch waste will not discharge into the stack less than 750 mm above the invert.

8. For buildings above five storeys, check that the ground floor appliances will discharge direct to drain or sub-stack, which may require venting. This will be independent of the main stacks from above.

9. For buildings above 20 storeys, check that the ground and first floor appliances will discharge into their own stacks separate from the floors above.

10. Check whether separate ventilation of branch pipes will be required (depends on the maximum number of connections, the length and slope of the branch discharge pipes, and whether traps or waterless traps are used).

11. Check that branch pipes serving a single appliance will be of a diameter at least the same as the appliance trap.

12. Check that if a pipe serves more than one appliance, and is unventilated, the diameter is at least the size shown in Table 2 of *Approved Document H1*. Note that Table A3 of *H1* provides additional minimal trap sizes and seal depths.

13. Check that the diameter of vertical discharge pipes meets the hydraulic capacities provided in Table 11 of *BS EN 12056-2* or Table 3 of *Approved Document H1*.

14. Check that an appropriately sized stack-ventilation pipe(s) will be provided.

15. For vacuum drainage systems check that the system is designed and sized in accordance with *BS EN 12109* (note that the static loss is in part a function of the pipe internal diameter).

16   FOUL WATER – BELOW GROUND DRAINAGE SYSTEM SIZING

Project title.. **Project No**.. **Design stage**.................

Engineer... **Revision No**................................... **Date**.............................

Checked by.. **Approved by**................................ **Date**.............................

Design inputs

✓ **Notes / Design file cross-reference**

- Discharge units (average discharge rate of a sanitary appliance)

  ☐

- Frequency factor (variable to take into account the frequency of use of sanitary appliances)

  ☐

- Above-ground drainage flows

  ☐

- Distance between one below ground drainage connection and the next

  ☐

- Sewer surcharge level, if any

  ☐

Design outputs

✓ **Notes / Design file cross-reference**

- Standard form recording results of calculations for submission for *Building Regulations* approval – See Table 3.14 of *CIBSE Guide G* for an example pro forma

  ☐

- Self cleansing velocities required

  ☐

- Fully detailed drainage drawings and specification indicating manhole positions, pipework layout, sizes, falls and levels, and invert levels

  ☐

Key design checks

✓ **Notes / Design file cross-reference**

- Check that the drains have enough capacity to carry the design flow. Note that capacity depends on the size and gradient of the pipe (hydraulic gradient)

  ☐

Project specific checks and notes

✓ **Notes / Design file cross-reference**

  ☐

  ☐

  ☐

16   FOUL WATER – BELOW GROUND DRAINAGE SYSTEM SIZING

Design inputs

- Discharge units (average discharge rate of a sanitary appliance)
- Frequency factor (variable to take into account the frequency of use of sanitary appliances)
- Above-ground drainage flows
- Distance between one below ground drainage connection and the next
- Sewer surcharge level, if any

Design information

- Number and type of sanitary appliances
- Location and layout of sanitary appliances within the building
- Kitchen equipment and any requirement for grease treatment
- Pump discharges
- Specialist discharges, such as sprinkler testing and trade waste discharges
- Final sewer (or drain) connection invert level/ site topography/ building finished floor levels

Design outputs

- Standard form recording results of calculations for submission for *Building Regulations* approval – See Table 3.14 of *CIBSE Guide G* for an example pro forma
- Self cleansing velocities required
- Fully detailed drainage drawings and specification indicating manhole positions, pipework layout, sizes, falls and levels, and invert levels

Key design checks

- Check that the drains have enough capacity to carry the design flow. Note that capacity depends on the size and gradient of the pipe (hydraulic gradient)

See also: Foul Water Below Ground Drainage Systems, Roof Drainage

---

DESIGN WATCHPOINTS

General watchpoints

1. Check that the total flow-rate from the building (or part of the building if relevant) has been estimated using the procedure detailed in *BS EN 12056-2*. (Predictions of simultaneous flows are made by the use of discharge units in conjunction with frequency factors.)

2. Be aware that discharge units are not interchangeable with demand units (the rates of filling and discharge differ).

3. Note that Table 5 of *Approved Document H1* provides design flow rates for different numbers of dwellings based on the calculation procedure provided in *BS EN 12056-2*.

4. Check that the drainage pipe gradient is adequate - Table 6 of *Approved Document H1* recommends minimum gradients for foul drains.

5. For general design work, check that the flow velocity will not be less than 0·6 m/s. Check that the velocity will not exceed 3 m/s in order to avoid scouring. Note that sometimes site topography may dictate steeper gradients than the usual calculated output leading to velocities exceeding 3 m/s. For combined foul and surface water drainage systems check that dry weather flow velocity will not be less than 0·6 m/s.

6. Check that the design is based on flow depths of 50-70%, backing-up and siphonage may occur at higher values.

7. Check that any pipe sizing software or sizing graphs and tables are based on the Colebrook-White flow equation.

8. For large developments check that the drains are sized to give a minimum self-cleansing velocity of 0·7 m/s (refer to *BS EN 752-4*, National Annex NA).

Available soon from BSRIA

Design checks for electrical services

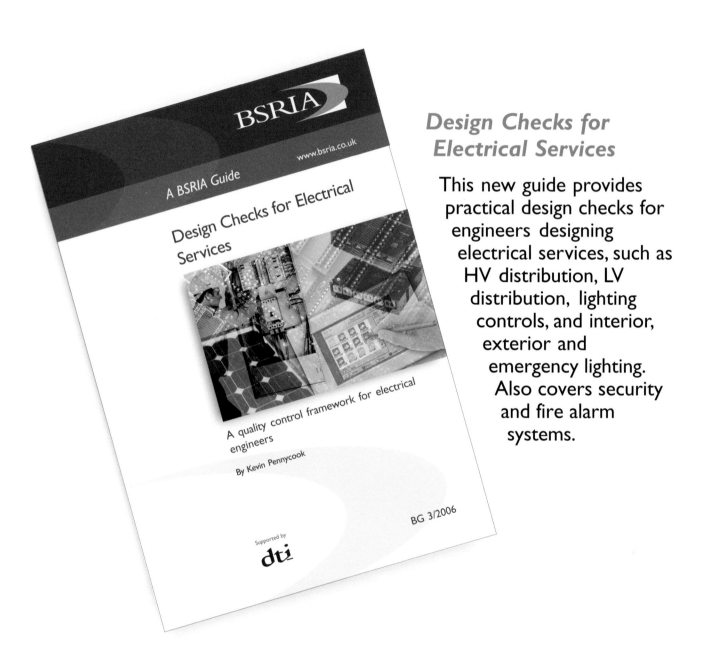

Design Checks for Electrical Services

This new guide provides practical design checks for engineers designing electrical services, such as HV distribution, LV distribution, lighting controls, and interior, exterior and emergency lighting. Also covers security and fire alarm systems.

Find this and other titles at

www.bsria.co.uk/bookshop

You can also order securely 24 hours a day, and sample before you buy!

SYSTEMS AND EQUIPMENT

17   COLD WATER STORAGE AND DISTRIBUTION

Project title .... **Project No**................................... **Design stage**..................

Engineer .... **Revision No**............................... **Date**..............................

Checked by .... **Approved by**............................ **Date**..............................

Design inputs

☑ **Notes / Design file cross-reference**

- Details of the application, such as the type of building and its function, number of occupants, number and type of sanitary fittings, and whether occupancy is permanent or transitory, and the balance between them ☐

- Period and hours of occupation and pattern of water use ☐

- Details of available water quantities and pressures from the water supply company (also any planned reductions in water pressure) ☐

- Water quality such as hardness (degrees Clark) and appropriate requirement for water treatment ☐

- Water storage capacity for client requirements, including any recommendations ☐

Design outputs

☑ **Notes / Design file cross-reference**

- Size, material options (such as plastics, galvanised steel, lined steel), location, fittings and thermal insulation of cisterns ☐

- Weight, type and supports required for cisterns ☐

- Requirements for access ☐

- Requirement for backflow-prevention devices ☐

- Cold water distribution network ☐

- See Design Outputs for Legionnaires' Disease – Cold Water Services ☐

Key design checks

☑ **Notes / Design file cross-reference**

- Systems have to comply with the *Water Supply (Water Fittings) Regulations 1999*, the *Water Byelaws 2000, Scotland* and the associated *Water Regulations Guide* ☐

- Systems should be designed in accordance with *BS 6700* and *BS EN 806-2* ☐

Project specific checks and notes

☑ **Notes / Design file cross-reference**

☐

☐

© BSRIA BG2/2006

17 COLD WATER STORAGE AND DISTRIBUTION

Design inputs

- Details of the application, such as the type of building and its function, number of occupants, number and type of sanitary fittings, and whether occupancy is permanent or transitory, and the balance between them
- Period and hours of occupation and pattern of water use
- Details of available water quantities and pressures from the water supply company (also any planned reductions in water pressure)
- Water quality such as hardness (degrees Clark) and appropriate requirement for water treatment
- Water storage capacity client requirements, including any recommendations

Design information

- Intended location of cistern and space allocation
- Location of water fittings
- Capacity for support for storage, (particularly if located in roof space), and in-ground detailing
- Quality of water to be stored, its hardness or acidity (this influences material of storage cistern and lifespan of cistern and associated components)
- Compatibility of cistern and system materials with intended water use

Design outputs

- Size, material options (including plastics, galvanised steel, and lined steel), location, fittings and thermal insulation of cisterns
- Weight, type and supports required for cisterns
- Requirements for access
- Requirement for backflow-prevention devices
- Cold water distribution network
- See Design Outputs for Legionnaires' Disease – Cold Water Services

Key design checks

- Systems have to comply with the *Water Supply (Water Fittings) Regulations 1999*, the *Water Byelaws 2000, Scotland* and the associated *Water Regulations Guide*
- Systems should be designed in accordance with *BS 6700* and *BS EN 806-2*

See also: Pipe Sizing– Cold and Hot Water Services, Hot Water Storage and Distribution, Legionnaires' Disease – Cold Water Services, Pressure Boosting of Water, Reclaimed Water Systems – General, Reclaimed Water Systems – Greywater, Reclaimed Water Systems - Rainwater

DESIGN WATCHPOINTS

Sizing and selection

1. Consider whether a gravity water system or a boosted water system is the more appropriate.
2. For a boosted water system, consider which of the following is the most appropriate: flooded suction to pressurise the cold water system to a high level break tank; suction lift to pressurise the cold water system to a high level break tank; flooded suction or suction lift to directly pressurise hot and cold water systems. (See Pressure Boosting of Water for further information.)
3. Consider any requirement for treatment.
4. Determine cold water storage requirements. See Tables 2.2 and 2.3 of *CIBSE Guide G* and Table 2 of *Plumbing Engineering Services Design-Guide: Section – Hot and Cold Water Supplies.*
5. Determine relevant fluid categories with regard to necessary backflow prevention measures. The risk of water being contaminated by backflow and the methods required to prevent this are detailed in the *Water Regulations Guide.* Check that these requirements are strictly adhered to.
6. Confirm with the architect the number of sanitary fittings based on the guidance provided by *BS 6465:Part 1.*
7. Consider likely client requirements for water storage capacity.
8. Check that cisterns over 1000 litre capacity are provided with compartments or a standby cistern in order to avoid interruption of the water supply when repairs or maintenance are carried out.
9. Check that cisterns over 1000 litre capacity are provided with a washout pipe located flush with the bottom of the cistern at its lowest point.
10. Check that the provision of overflows and warning pipes for cisterns comply with the *Water Supply (Water Fittings) Regulations* and the *Water Byelaws 2000, Scotland.*
11. Consider how best to minimise noise. Check that pipes are not fixed rigidly to lightweight panels. Install pipes within substantial enclosures. Consider the location of pipes in relation to noise-sensitive areas. Take care in the design of pipework layouts to minimise the possibility of cavitation occurring by ensuring that low pressure/high velocity situations are avoided in the pipework layouts. Consider the different approaches to alleviate water hammer and select the most appropriate solution. Transmission of pump and motor noise can be reduced by the use of flexible connections and anti-vibration mountings.
12. Consider the risk of frost damage. The location of pipes, cisterns and system components must be considered. If frost damage is possible, protection should be provided in accordance with *BS 6700* and the *Water Regulations Guide.*
13. Check that structural requirements for weight loadings have been allowed for by the structural engineer.
14. Consider requirements for cistern base/support pier requirements according to the type of storage system selected.
15. Consider connections for level switches/temperature sensor points.

16. Allow for pressure-reduction valves where appropriate.
17. Consider the risk of bimetallic corrosion where dissimilar metals are being connected.
18. For hospitals and other healthcare buildings, check that the requirements of *HTM 2027* are met.

Installation, operation and control

19. Check that all pipework/appliances and controls do not obstruct users.
20. Check that pipework and fixings are enclosed to deter vandalism and avoid accidental damage.
21. Check that services are colour banded in accordance with *BS 1710.*
22. Consider sterilisation of the system in accordance with *BS 6700.*
23. Check that suitable identification of services are provided.
24. Check that provision is made for an operating and maintenance manual and/or incorporation of operating details in the building log book.
25. Consider any requirements for bunds.
26. Check requirements for electrical earthing and bonding in accordance with *BS 7671.*
27. When pipes are to be installed in ducts, check that the requirements of *BS 8313* are followed.
28. Consider requirements for the protective coating of pipework, such as if bedded in corrosive materials such as concrete or contaminated land.
29. Check that the system will be commissioned in accordance with *CIBSE Commissioning Code W* and *BSRIA AG 2/89.3* where relevant.

Access and maintenance

30. Check that sufficient access to cisterns for installation, commissioning, testing and maintenance is provided. Check that cisterns allow reasonable access to the inside so that it may be easily inspected and cleaned, and so that the float operated valve (or other comparable device) may be easily adjusted, repaired or renewed.
31. Check that cisterns will be fitted with a rigid, close fitting and securely fixed cover that is not airtight but excludes light and insects.
32. Check that all valves, including any backflow prevention devices, are readily accessible for examination, commissioning, testing and maintenance.
33. For large storage cisterns check internal/external access ladders are provided where necessary Consider hand railing around tops of tall cisterns where there is a danger of falling from height.
34. Consider requirements for future pipe repainting.

Economics

35. When costing, consideration should be given to both the cost of materials and fittings and different methods of installation.
36. Consider life cycle costs based on storage vessel material, maintenance, cleaning and the expected use and life of the building.
37. Consider the likely influence of water quality on the lifespan of the system and the economic benefit of water treatment.

© BSRIA BG2/2006

18   HOT WATER STORAGE AND DISTRIBUTION

Project title.. **Project No**... **Design stage**...................

Engineer.. **Revision No**.. **Date**...............................

Checked by... **Approved by**....................................... **Date**...............................

Design inputs

- Number of occupants, and the split between permanent and transitory occupancy

- Period and hours of occupation and pattern of hot water use

- The client's requirement for hot water storage

- Water quality, including hardness, and the appropriate requirement for water treatment

Notes / Design file cross-reference

Design outputs

- Schematics showing the installation of hot water storage vessel(s) showing connections and outlets

- Schedule of hot water storage vessel sizes, capacity, recovery period, primary heat source, working pressures (primary and secondary), whether vented or un-vented, and weights at full capacity

- Hot water distribution network

- Control requirements

- Requirement for backflow prevention

- See Design Outputs for Legionnaires' Disease – Hot Water Services

- Assessment of primary heat-source loads, including whether gas or electric

Notes / Design file cross-reference

Key design checks

- Check that the hot water storage vessel system is correctly sized

- Check that the supply and return pipes are correctly sized

- Systems have to comply with the *Water Supply (Water Fittings) Regulations 1999*, the *Water Bylaws 2000 Scotland* and the associated *Water Regulations Guide*

- Systems should be designed in accordance with *BS 6700* and *BS EN 806-2*

- Design in accordance with *HSC ACOP L8* – See Legionnaires' Disease – Hot Water Services

Notes / Design file cross-reference

Project specific checks and notes

Notes / Design file cross-reference

18 HOT WATER STORAGE AND DISTRIBUTION

Design inputs

- Number of occupants, and the split between permanent and transitory occupancy
- Period and hours of occupation and pattern of hot water use
- The client's requirement for hot water storage
- Water quality, including hardness, and the appropriate requirement for water treatment

Design information

- Details of building type and function
- Locations and space available for installation
- Information on availability of gas and electric supply for point of use water heating
- Information on available primary heat sources, such as flow temperatures and flow rate for low pressure hot water
- Location of water fittings

Design outputs

- Schematics showing the installation of hot water storage vessel(s) showing connections and outlets

See also: Pipe Sizing– Cold and Hot Water Services, Cold Water Storage and Distribution, Legionnaires' Disease – Hot Water Services, Pressure Boosting of Water

- Schedule of hot water storage vessel sizes, capacity, recovery period, primary heat source, working pressures (primary and secondary), whether vented or un-vented, and weights at full capacity
- Hot water distribution network
- Control requirements
- Requirement for backflow prevention
- See Design Outputs for Legionnaires' Disease – Hot Water Services
- Assessment of primary heat source loads, and whether gas or electric

Key design checks

- Check that the hot water storage vessel system is correctly sized
- Check that the supply and return pipes are correctly sized
- Systems have to comply with the *Water Supply (Water Fittings) Regulations 1999*, the *Water Bylaws 2000, Scotland* and the associated *Water Regulations Guide*
- Systems should be designed in accordance with *BS 6700* and *BS EN 806-2*
- Design in accordance with *HSC ACOP L8* – See Legionnaires' Disease – Hot Water Services

DESIGN WATCHPOINTS

Sizing and selection

1. Consider whether hot water storage or instantaneous water heating is the most appropriate. For instantaneous water heating, decide between multi-outlet or single outlet.
2. When determining hot water storage capacity, consider both design consumption rate and the recovery rate. Table 2.10 of *CIBSE Guide* G provides guidance for a range of applications.
3. Consider any requirement for water treatment.
4. Determine relevant fluid categories with regard to necessary backflow prevention measures. The risk of water being contaminated by backflow and the methods required to prevent this are detailed in the *Water Regulations Guide*. Check that these requirements are strictly adhered to.
5. Check that unvented hot water storage systems comply with *Approved Document G3*.
6. Confirm with the Architect the number of sanitary fittings based on the guidance provided by *BS 645:Part 1*.
7. Consider the risk of frost damage and appropriate protection measures.
8. Consider the risk of bimetallic corrosion where dissimilar metals are to be connected.
9. Consider the choice of pipework. Decide between copper, stainless steel, polybutylene, PVC-C or similar.
10. Consider the use of a local water conditioner.
11. Consider any requirement for multiple storage tanks where interruption to the supply due to plant failure cannot be tolerated, such as in hospitals and industrial processes.
12. Consider the use of instantaneous hot water, such as direct gas-fired water heaters and plate heat-exchangers.

Installation, operation and control

13. Check that all pipework/appliances and controls do not obstruct users.
14. Check that pipework and fixings are enclosed to deter vandalism and avoid accidental damage.
15. Check that services are colour banded in accordance with *BS 1710*.
16. Check that suitable identification of services will be provided.
17. Check that provision is made for an operating and maintenance manual and/or incorporation of operating details in the building log book.
18. Check requirements for electrical earthing and bonding in accordance with *BS 7671*.

19. When pipes are to be installed in ducts, check that the requirements of *BS 8313* are followed.
20. Check that there will be sufficient space for safe installation and maintenance of the calorifier and associated plant and equipment.
21. Check that the system will be commissioned in accordance with *CIBSE Commissioning Code W* and *BSRIA AG 2/89.3*.
22. Check that the normal operating storage water temperature will not exceed 65°C.
23. Check that levels of chlorine (for sterilisation purposes) will not exceed that specified in *HSE ACOP L8*.
24. Check that adequately-sized expansion vessels are provided for unvented hot water storage systems when required.
25. Check that thermostatic mixer valves are fitted to outlets. If not, check that a warning sign stating 'Very Hot Water' will be fitted on the wall at the appliance.
26. Check that outlet temperatures meet the occupant's needs. Lower temperatures are required in hospitals, schools, nursing homes, and retirement homes.
27. For hospitals and other healthcare buildings check that the requirements of *HTM 2027* are met.
28. Where necessary check that adequate provision will be provided to monitor through the building management system.

Access and maintenance

29. Check that pipework to the services will be sited where possible to enable inspection and repair.
30. Provide sufficient flushing and chemical cleaning supply points and drains.
31. Check that drain points will be installed at low points.

Economics

32. Consider the likely influence of water quality on the lifespan of the system and the economic benefit of water treatment.
33. Consider life-cycle costs based on equipment cost, maintenance, cleaning and the expected use and life of the building.
34. When costing, consideration should be given to both the cost of materials and fittings and different methods of installation.

19   LEGIONNAIRES' DISEASE – COLD WATER SERVICES

Project title .... **Project No** .... **Design stage** ....

Engineer .... **Revision No** .... **Date** ....

Checked by .... **Approved by** .... **Date** ....

Design inputs

- Cold water demand and patterns of use

- Likely maximum interruption of mains water supply

- Criticality of water supply

- Results of *legionella* risk assessment

- Options for water treatment, such as ionisation, iodine and chlorine dioxide

Notes / Design file cross-reference

Design outputs

- Insulation requirements for cold water pipework

- Requirements for additional water treatment

- Specification of fittings and materials

- Design of system branches

- See Design Outputs for Cold Water Storage and Distribution

Notes / Design file cross-reference

Key design checks

- Avoid tepid water conditions (Storage/distribution temperatures in the range 20 – 45°C will support significant colonies of bacteria.)

- Design in accordance with *HSC ACOP L8 – The control of legionella bacteria in water systems* and *CIBSE TM 13 – Minimising the risk of legionnaires' disease*

- Systems have to comply with the *Water Supply (Water Fittings) Regulations 1999* and the *Water Byelaws 2000, Scotland*

- Systems should be designed in accordance with *BS 6700* and *BS EN 806-2*

Notes / Design file cross-reference

Project specific checks and notes

Notes / Design file cross-reference

© BSRIA BG2/2006

19 LEGIONNAIRES' DISEASE – COLD WATER SERVICES

Design inputs

- Cold water demand and patterns of use
- Likely maximum interruption of mains water supply
- Criticality of water supply
- Results of *legionella* risk assessment
- Options for water treatment, such as ionisation, iodine and chlorine dioxide

Design information

- Intended location of cistern(s) and space allocation
- Location of water fittings
- Location of hot water pipes and other sources of heat

See also: Cold Water Storage and Distribution, Hot Water Storage and Distribution

Design outputs

- Insulation requirements for cold water pipework
- Requirements for additional water treatment
- Specification of fittings and materials
- Design of system branches
- See Design Outputs for Cold Water Storage and Distribution

Key design checks

- Avoid tepid water conditions (Storage/distribution temperatures in the range 20 – 45°C will support significant colonies of bacteria.)
- Design in accordance with *HSC ACOP L8 – The control of legionella bacteria in water systems* and *CIBSE TM 13 – Minimising the risk of legionnaires' disease*
- Systems have to comply with the *Water Supply (Water Fittings) Regulations 1999* and the *Water Byelaws 2000, Scotland*
- Systems should be designed in accordance with *BS 6700* and *BS EN 806-2*

DESIGN WATCHPOINTS

Sizing and selection

1. Cold-water piping should be insulated and kept away from sources of heat such as hot pipes and ductwork. Temperature rises due to heat sources should be limited to 2°C.
2. Water services cisterns should comply with the *Water Supply (Water Fittings) Regulations 1999* and the *Water Byelaws 2000, Scotland*.
3. Cisterns should be provided with a close-fitting removable cover to protect against ingress of dirt. Overflow and vents should be protected by insect-proof screens.
4. Cistern should be sited in a cool place and protected from extremes of temperature by thermal insulation. Where the cistern is installed inside a roof space, the roof should be well ventilated.
5. Design storage capacity based on the likely maximum duration of interruption of mains supply should typically be less than one working day. Table 2.3 in *CIBSE Guide G* provides appropriate guidance. Longer storage times may require additional treatment and provision for regular or continuous chlorination or other means of disinfection such as chlorine dioxide dosage of ionisation. See *HSC ACOP L8* for further guidance.
6. Check that cistern inlet and outlet connections are arranged such that stagnation of the stored water will not occur.
7. Multiple linked storage-tanks should be avoided where possible because of difficulties due to possible unequal flow rates and possible stagnation. Note that it is essential not to oversize storage tanks.
8. Fittings and materials for sealants, gaskets and washers should be selected from the *Water Fittings and Materials Directory* published by the WRAS. Materials such as natural rubber, hemp, linseed oil-based jointing compounds and fibre washers should not be used.
9. Locate water fittings with high usage at the end of system branches to ensure the best possible water throughput and to minimise stagnation.
10. Check that systems are colour banded in accordance with *BS 1710*.
11. Consider sterilisation of the system in accordance with *BS 6700*.
12. As an alternative to the temperature regime method, consider the use of approaches such as chemical dosing with supplementary chlorine dioxide, and ionisation treatment with silver and copper electrodes.

Installation, operation and control

13. The temperature of cold water at a tap should not exceed 20°C after the water has been running for two minutes.
14. Provide a bottom outlet from cisterns (where practical) to reduce sediment retention in the cistern bottom.
15. For existing cisterns use plastic liners where appropriate rather than painting the inside.

Access and maintenance

16. Small cisterns should be provided with a removable cover for inspection of the cistern and maintenance of the float-operated valve.
17. Larger systems (> 1000 litres) should be provided with a hinged cover for the maintenance of float-operated valves and similar additional hatches for inspection.
18. Provision should be made for cleaning internal surfaces of cisterns without major interruption. Where continuous cold-water service is required consider the use of a small break-tank sized for the maximum draw-off rate. This will allow the supply to be taken temporarily from the break-tank whenever maintenance is needed on the main storage cistern.
19. Avoid internally-flanged sectional cisterns, as they are difficult to clean.
20. Provide adequate access to strainers, water softeners and filters.
21. Accumulator vessels on hot and cold-water services should be fitted with diaphragms that are accessible for cleaning. Two pipe models are preferable as they provide a through-flow.
22. Pipework should be easy to inspect so that the thermal insulation can be checked to confirm that it is in position and undisturbed.
23. Provide information for the operating and maintenance manual and water quality monitoring log book.
24. Provide an indication of factors that will influence the frequency of maintenance actions.

Economics

25. Conduct a component option-appraisal taking into account capital costs and maintenance costs in the context of managing the risk.
26. Consider the use of remote real time monitoring, such as monitoring using a building management system.

20 LEGIONNAIRES' DISEASE – HOT WATER SERVICES

Project title .... **Project No** .... **Design stage** ....

Engineer .... **Revision No** .... **Date** ....

Checked by .... **Approved by** .... **Date** ....

Design inputs

- Hot water demand and patterns of use ☐
- Results of *legionella* risk assessment ☐
- Options for water treatment, such as ionisation, chlorine dioxide or iodine dosage ☐

✓ Notes / Design file cross-reference

Design outputs

- Size, location, thermal insulation and access for calorifiers ☐
- Insulation requirements for pipework ☐
- Requirements for water treatment ☐
- Specification for fittings and materials ☐
- Design of distribution system including size and route of pipes ☐
- See Design Outputs for Hot Water Storage and Distribution ☐

✓ Notes / Design file cross-reference

Key design checks

- Design in accordance with *HSC ACOP L8 – The control of legionella bacteria in water systems* and *CIBSE TM 13 – Minimising the risk of legionnaires' disease* ☐
- Systems have to comply with the *Water Supply (Water Fittings) Regulations 1999* and the *Water Byelaws 2000, Scotland* ☐
- Systems should be designed in accordance with *BS 6700 and BS EN 806-2* ☐
- Consider the use of supplementary treatments such as chlorine dioxide dosage and silver/copper ionisation where treatment control may be poor and would present consistent operational difficulties ☐
- Consider which type of system is most appropriate: pumped flow and return; non-recirculating trace heated system; or point-of-use water heaters ☐

✓ Notes / Design file cross-reference

Project specific checks and notes

☐
☐
☐

✓ Notes / Design file cross-reference

© BSRIA BG2/2006

20 LEGIONNAIRES' DISEASE – HOT WATER SERVICES

Design inputs

- Hot water demand and patterns of use
- Results of *legionella* risk assessment
- Options for water treatment, such as ionisation, chlorine dioxide and iodine dosage

Design information

- Building use, such as office, hospital or school
- Intended location of taps and other outlets
- Intended location of calorifier and space allocation
- High-risk components

Design outputs

- Size, location, thermal insulation and access for calorifiers
- Insulation requirements for pipework
- Requirements for water treatment
- Specification for fittings and materials
- Design of distribution system including size and route of pipes
- See Design Outputs for Hot Water Storage and Distribution

Key design checks

- Design in accordance with *HSC ACOP L8 – The control of legionella bacteria in water systems* and *CIBSE TM 13 – Minimising the risk of legionnaires' disease*
- Systems have to comply with the *Water Supply (Water Fittings) Regulations 1999* and the *Water Byelaws 2000, Scotland*
- Systems should be designed in accordance with *BS 6700* and *BS EN 806-2*
- Consider the use of supplementary treatments such as chlorine dioxide dosage, iodine dosage and silver/copper ionisation where treatment control may be poor and would present consistent operational difficulties
- Consider which type of system is most appropriate: pumped flow and return; non-recirculating trace heated system; or point-of-use water heaters

See also: Cold Water Storage and Distribution, Hot Water Storage and Distribution, Legionnaires' Disease – Cold Water Services

DESIGN WATCHPOINTS

Sizing and selection

1. Check that the distribution pipework design enables the water at taps to reach 50°C within one minute of turning on the tap (check that thermostatic mixing valves (TMVs) are installed with temperature test nipples).

2. Avoid pipework deadlegs and long runs from which there is only an occasional draw-off.

3. Check that the calorifier will be capable of maintaining a supply temperature of 60°C under normal operating conditions including times of peak demand.

4. Check that the design outlet temperature is based on the extent of the distribution system, storage temperature, pipework heat loss, and demand patterns.

5. For pumped flow and return systems, the pump performance should be selected to offset the losses from the distribution pipework circuit with a given temperature drop.

6. For non-recirculating systems, determine whether hot water maintenance tape (electric trace heating) is required to ensure draw-off outflows of 50°C within one minute of opening the outlets.

7. Calorifier design should ensure reasonably uniform bulk storage temperatures throughout. Consider the use of a recirculation (or shunt) pump to eliminate temperature stratification within the calorifier. Provide thermal insulation on the underside of calorifiers that incorporate a recirculation pump.

8. Check that calorifiers are capable of occasionally being heated to 70°C throughout for pasteurisation purposes.

9. Consider the risk to susceptible occupants posed by reverse flow through the return circulation pipework under draw-off. This can be minimised by fitting a non-return valve and/or pump on the return part of the recirculation circuit adjacent to the calorifier.

10. Provide thermostatic mixing valves in appropriate applications: TMV2 in public areas and TMV3 in hospitals, care homes and schools. Check that TMVs will be sited as close as possible to the draw-off point. Check that where a single TMV serves more that one outlet, the outlets will be used frequently or thoroughly flushed regularly.

11. Check that showers (excluding safety showers) will not be fitted where they are likely to be used less than once a week.

12. Check that flow and return pipes are insulated.

13. Fittings and materials for sealants, gaskets and washers should be selected from the *Water Fittings and Materials Directory* published by the Water Research Centre. Materials such as natural rubber, hemp, linseed oil-based jointing compounds and fibre washers should not be used.

14. Check that calorifiers will have adequate thermal insulation.

Installation, operation and control

15. The storage temperature, controlled from a thermostat, should be 60°C.

16. Thermometer or immersion pockets should be fitted on the flow and return to the calorifier and in the base of the calorifier in addition to those required for control.

17. Prolonged storage time at high temperatures is beneficial as it aids pasteurisation effectiveness.

18. Consider the need for warning notices warning of possible high temperature. Check that water temperatures will not exceed 55°C at taps (lower temperatures are applicable for certain applications such as health care and schools where occupants are vulnerable to scalding).

19. Where a recirculation/shunt pump is used in conjunction with a calorifier in order to avoid temperature differences (stratification) ensure that the pump is only switched on during periods of no demand. The pump should not be running during water draw-off as temperature stratification will help to maintain the design supply temperature.

20. Check that the hot water circuit(s) will be correctly balanced. Consider the use of double regulating valves and thermal balancing valves.

21. Check that the commissioning requirements of *HSC L8* will be met.

22. Check that services will be colour banded in accordance with *BS 1710*.

Access and maintenance

23. Calorifiers should have easy access for inspection, draining, dismantling and cleaning. A large drain or dump valve at the lowest point is required to allow rapid draining and removal of sludge. Specify calorifier designs that minimise the scope for the entrapment of sludge.

24. Accumulator vessels on pressurised systems should be fitted with diaphragms that are accessible for cleaning. Two-pipe models are preferable to ensure through flow.

25. Pipework should be easy to inspect so that the thermal insulation can be checked to confirm that it is in position and undisturbed.

26. Provide information for the operating and maintenance manual and water quality monitoring logbook.

27. Provide an indication of factors that will influence the frequency of maintenance actions.

Economics

28. Conduct a component option appraisal taking into account capital costs and maintenance costs in the context of managing the risk.

29. Consider the use of remote real time monitoring, such as monitoring using a building management system.

21 PRESSURE BOOSTING OF WATER

Project title.. **Project No**......................... **Design stage**................

Engineer... **Revision No** .... **Date**..........................

Checked by... **Approved by** .... **Date**..........................

Design inputs

- Pressure required (in bar) at highest point in the system

- Design flow rates (maximum, design and minimum flow rates) and diversity

- Temperature of water (maximum, design, minimum)

- Interface requirements with the building management system (BMS)

- Type of application (raising head, providing flow, maintaining a pressure)

- Availability of electrical supply and loads required

Notes / Design file cross-reference

Design outputs

- Selection and number of pumps, such as, fixed, variable, and multistage

- Selection of pressurisation unit and size of expansion vessel (could be done in conjunction with packaged booster pump system manufacturer)

- Definition of switching pumps 'on' and 'off' to meet design criteria (based on flow switch, pressure switches or transmitter)

- Pump controls (duty, assist and standby)

Notes / Design file cross-reference

Key design checks

- Verify that the net pressure suction head (NPSH) calculation has been carried out, especially for high temperature applications

- If pumped water will also be used for drinking water, verify that components meet the *Water Regulations*

- Consider the use of a jockey pump to supply the system's minimum requirements (alternatively consider variable speed pumps)

- For suction-lift systems, verify that the water in the suction pipework will be prevented from draining back into the cistern, such as by a foot valve

- For unvented hot water systems, verify that due consideration has been given to over-pressure from expansion

Notes / Design file cross-reference

© BSRIA BG2/2006

21 PRESSURE BOOSTING OF WATER

Project title.. **Project No**... **Design stage**...................

Engineer.. **Revision No** .... **Date** ....

Checked by... **Approved by** .... **Date** ....

Key design checks (cont.)

- Where hot water systems and cold water systems are combined, check that single check-valves are installed between the hot water system and the cold water system to avoid migration between the two

- For a hot water system, verify that an expansion vessel or accumulator is installed on the cold feed (or an integral expansion facility on the cylinder)

- For a hot water system, verify that an expansion vessel, and temperature and pressure relief valves will be fitted to protect the water heater from possible failure or rupture

Project specific checks and notes

✓ **Notes / Design file cross-reference**

✓ **Notes / Design file cross-reference**

© BSRIA BG2/2006

21 PRESSURE BOOSTING OF WATER

Design inputs

- Pressure required (in bar) at highest point in the system
- Design flow rates (maximum, design and minimum flow rates) and diversity
- Temperature of water (maximum, design, minimum)
- Interface requirements with building management system
- Type of application (raising head, providing flow, maintaining a pressure)
- Availability of electrical supply and loads required

Design information

- Pipework routing
- Pipework material (such as copper, plastic, and stainless steel)
- Pressure drops across the system and the residual static head required
- Inverter drive or staged pumps and jockey pump

Design outputs

- Selection and number of pumps, such as fixed, variable, or multistage
- Selection of pressurisation unit and size of expansion vessel (could be done in conjunction with the manufacturer or the packaged booster pump system)
- Definition of switching pumps 'on' and 'off' to meet design criteria. (Based on flow switch, pressure switches or transmitter.)
- Pump controls (duty, assist and standby)

Key design checks

- Verify that the net pressure suction head (NPSH) calculation has been carried out, especially for high temperature applications
- If pumped water will also be used for drinking water, verify that components meet the *Water Regulations*
- Consider the use of a jockey pump to supply the system's minimum requirements (alternatively consider variable speed pumps)
- For suction-lift systems, verify that the water in the suction pipework will be prevented from draining back into the cistern, such as by a foot valve
- For unvented hot water systems, verify that due consideration has been given to over-pressure from expansion
- Where the hot water system and the cold water systems are combined, check that single check-valves are installed between the hot water system and the cold water system to avoid migration between the two
- For the hot water systems, verify that an expansion vessel or accumulator is installed on the cold feed (or an integral expansion facility on the cylinder)
- For the hot water system, verify that an expansion vessel, temperature and pressure relief valves will be fitted to protect the water heater from possible failure or rupture

See also: Mains Water Availability, Cold Water Storage and Distribution

DESIGN WATCHPOINTS

Sizing and selection

1. Verify that the (smallest) pump and lowest viable setting of inverter (if applicable) will match the minimum demand.
2. If the system includes a bypass, verify that this has been included within the documentation.
3. Check that the maximum pressure for the system matches the maximum possible delivery pressure of the pumps (from the pump curve).
4. Verify that for each pump operating mode there is a minimum one minute running between switching on and off. (Check with the pump manufacturer.)
5. When a break tank feeds the pump(s), ensure that a low level cut-out will disable the pump.
6. Check that pump controls include automatic rotation of duty and standby pumps, adjustable start-time delays, adjustable run-on delays, 'hand/off/auto' control for each pump, low level water cut-out, pump running fault indication and an audible alarm and interface with the building management system.
7. Check that pumps that have a fault are automatically omitted from the control sequence.
8. Consider how water level and pump failure alarms will be provided that ensure identification by the user.
9. Verify with the packaged booster pump system manufacturer on the sizing of the accumulator vessel.
10. Consider the use of hydraulic shock arrestors on risers and end of runs.
11. If fixed speed pumps are selected, check that pump closed, valve-head pressure will not over-pressurise the system.
12. Consider problems associated with closed valve heads.
13. Consider the volume of the hydraulic accumulator as this will reduce hydraulic shock.
14. Verify that safe discharge will be available for pressure and temperature relief drain or expansion valve drain.

Installation, operation and control

15. In the event that pump skids are procured check that allowance has been made for its ingress into the building and final location.
16. Verify that pumps have non-return valves fitted on the discharge side.
17. Check if isolation valves have been fitted to each pump on the discharge and suction side for isolation purposes during maintenance.
18. Check that the system includes pressure indication on the discharge side. (Optional on the inlet.)
19. Pumps (suction and discharge) should be fitted with anti-vibration couplings (WRAS approved) to minimise vibration from the pump(s) to the pipework system.
20. Consider the installation of anti-vibration mountings for installing the pump and skid base plate to the structure. (Consult manufacturer for details.)
21. Verify if the isolating stop valve and drain valves will be fitted to the pressure vessel and accumulator.

Access and maintenance

22. Consider the use of strainers on the inlet to the pumps to protect them from damage from particulates in the pipework system.

Economics

23. Check that consideration has been taken of, Enhanced Capital Allowance for variable frequency inverters versus 'on/off' control and use of bypasses and double regulating valves.
24. Consider supplying low level demand points direct from the incoming mains.
25. Consider whole-life costs of different systems and pump options – particularly in terms of energy use and risk of component failure.

22 DRINKING WATER SYSTEMS

Project title... **Project No**.. **Design stage**...................

Engineer.. **Revision No**.. **Date**..............................

Checked by.. **Approved by**.................................... **Date**..............................

Design inputs

Notes / Design file cross-reference

- Details of the application, such as the type of building and its function, number of occupants and sanitary appliances and whether occupancy is permanent or transitory, and the balance between the two ☐

- Period and hours of occupation and pattern of water use ☐

- Details of available water quantities, water quality and pressures from the water supply company ☐

Design outputs

Notes / Design file cross-reference

- Mains water distribution network ☐

- Requirement for backflow-prevention devices ☐

Key design checks

Notes / Design file cross-reference

- Check for compliance with the *Water Supply (Water Fittings) Regulations 1999, Water Byelaws 2000, Scotland* and the associated *Water Regulations Guide* ☐

- Systems should be designed in accordance with *BS 6700 and BS EN 806-2* ☐

- Follow the guidance provided in the *Plumbing Engineering Services Design Guide* (Institute of Plumbing and Heating Engineering) ☐

Project specific checks and notes

Notes / Design file cross-reference

☐
☐
☐

22 DRINKING WATER SYSTEMS

Design inputs

- Details of the application, such as the type of building and its function, number of occupants and sanitary appliances and whether occupancy is permanent or transitory, and the balance between the two
- Period and hours of occupation and pattern of water use
- Details of available water quantities and pressures from the water supply company and water quality

Design information

- Intended location of all possible drinking water outlets such as sinks, basins, and vending machines

See also: Contamination Prevention, Pipe Sizing – Cold and Hot Water Services, Cold Water Storage and Distribution, Legionnaires' Disease – Cold Water Services, Pressure Boosting of Water.

Design outputs

- Mains water distribution network
- Requirement for backflow prevention devices

Key design checks

- Check for compliance with the *Water Supply (Water Fittings) Regulations 1999* and the *Water Byelaws 2000, Scotland* and the associated *Water Regulations Guide*
- Systems should be designed in accordance with *BS 6700 and BS EN 806-2*
- Follow the guidance provided in the *Plumbing Engineering Services Design Guide* (Institute of Plumbing and Heating Engineering)

DESIGN WATCHPOINTS

Sizing and selection

1. Consider whether a direct mains-water system or a boosted water system is the more appropriate.
2. For a boosted water system, consider which of the following is the most appropriate: flooded suction to pressurise the cold water system to a high level break tank; suction lift to pressurise the cold water system to a high level break tank; flooded suction or suction lift, fed from a low-level break tank, to directly pressurise cold water systems.
3. Consider pipework layout in relation to drinking water outlets so as to avoid long dead legs to isolated fittings. Check that high volume fittings are downstream of less frequently used fittings such as a sink fitted after the branch for a vending machine or drinking fountain.
4. Consider whether pressure-reducing valves and flow limiters are to be fitted where the mains water pressure and flow may be in excess of that required by a particular drinking water component such as for drinks vending machine or water cooler.
5. Consider if any form of water filtering or conditioning is required and what form this will take.
6. Check that branch connections to drinking water outlets are kept as short as possible to avoid stagnation.
7. Check that pipework is adequately insulated to prevent a rise in temperature of the drinking water supply in accordance with *Water Supply (Water Fittings) Regulation 1999* and the *Water Byelaws 2000, Scotland* and *BS 6700*. Where pipework is grouped and banked vertically, check that drinking water pipework is fixed below any hot water or heating pipework to reduce heat gain.
8. Determine relevant fluid categories with regard to necessary backflow prevention measures. The risk of water being contaminated by backflow and the methods required to prevent this are detailed in the *Water Regulations Guide*. Check that these requirements are strictly adhered to. (See Contamination Prevention.)

9. Consider how best to minimise noise. Check that pipes are not fixed rigidly to lightweight panels. Install pipes within substantial and reasonably airtight ducts or enclosures. Take care in the design of pipework layouts to minimise the possibility of cavitation occurring by ensuring that low pressure, high velocity situations are avoided in the pipework layouts. Consider the different approaches to alleviate water hammer and select the most appropriate solution. Transmission of pump and motor noise can be reduced by the use of flexible connections and anti-vibration mountings.
10. Consider the risk of frost damage. The location of pipes, cisterns and system components must be considered. If frost damage is possible, protection should be provided in accordance with *BS 6700* and the *Water Regulations Guide*.
11. Check services are colour banded in accordance with *BS 1710*.
12. Consider sterilisation of the system in accordance with *BS 6700*.

Installation, operation and control

13. Check that all pipework, appliances and controls do not obstruct users.
14. Check that pipework and fixings are enclosed to deter vandalism and avoid accidental damage.

Access and maintenance

15. Check that all valves, including any backflow prevention devices, are readily accessible for examination, commissioning, testing and maintenance. Check that any covers are fixed by removable fittings.

Economics

16. Consider whole life costs particularly where filtering and conditioning are likely to incur significant servicing, maintenance and component replacement costs.

© BSRIA BG2/2006

23   WATER TREATMENT

Project title .... **Project No** .... **Design stage** ....

Engineer .... **Revision No** .... **Date** ....

Checked by .... **Approved by** .... **Date** ....

Design inputs

✓ **Notes / Design file cross-reference**

- Details of local water supply quality: physical characteristics (such as colour, odour, taste, and ph) and chemical characteristics (for example inorganic and organic parameters)

☐

- Details of proposed systems within the building that require a treated water supply, plus information on the required quality of water and system volumes

☐

Design outputs

✓ **Notes / Design file cross-reference**

- Type of water treatment required

☐

- Capacity of selected water treatment

☐

Key design checks

✓ **Notes / Design file cross-reference**

- Comply with the requirements of the *Water Supply (Water Fittings) Regulations 1999* (the *Water Byelaws 2000* in Scotland) and the associated *Water Regulations Guide* are met

☐

- Comply with the requirements of *BS 6700 and BS EN 806-2*

☐

- Comply with the requirements of *HSC L8*

☐

Project specific checks and notes

✓ **Notes / Design file cross-reference**

☐

☐

☐

23 WATER TREATMENT

Design inputs

- Details of local water supply quality: physical characteristics (such as colour, odour, taste, and ph) and chemical characteristics (for example inorganic and organic parameters)
- Details of proposed systems within the building that require a treated water supply, plus information on the required quality of water and system volumes

Design information

- Details of all system components and equipment including details of composition, such as materials

See also: Legionnaires' Disease – Cold Water Services, Legionnaires Disease' – Hot Water Services

Design outputs

- Type of water treatment required
- Capacity of selected water treatment

Key design checks

- Comply with the requirements of the *Water Supply (Water Fittings) Regulations 1999* (the *Water Byelaws 2000* in Scotland) and the associated *Water Regulations Guide* are met
- Comply with the requirements of *BS 6700* and *BS EN 806-2*
- Comply with the requirements of *HSC L8*

DESIGN WATCHPOINTS

Sizing and selection

1. Consider the following options:
   - Filtration
   - Electromagnetic conditioning
   - Water softening
   - Ultraviolet light
   - Reverse osmosis
   - Chlorine dioxide
   - De-calcification
   - Vortex filter
   - Ionisation.

2. For the protection against *legionella* consider: full temperature regime, ultraviolet radiation, copper/silver ionisation, and ozone treatment. Note that the *HSE Approved Code of Practice (L8)* on the control of legionellosis risk recommends that a full temperature regime is the preferred option for domestic hot water systems.

3. For water softeners consider: ion exchange, reverse osmosis, or distillation.

4. Consider the use of a chemical water conditioner for the reduction of levels of calcium and magnesium.

5. Consider that scale formation can be reduced through the use of a physical water conditioner such as an electronic, electrolytic, magnetic or electromagnetic device.

6. For swimming pool, check that the water treatment system is designed in accordance with the PWTAG *Swimming Pool Water Treatment and Quality Standards*. Check that water inlets/outlets, drains, skimmers, and overflow channels comply with the requirements of *BS EN 13451-3*.

7. For water features and fountains consider the following treatment options:
   - Bleed/top-up
   - Filtration
   - Sodium hypochlorite solution
   - Electro chlorination
   - Bromination
   - Ultraviolet light
   - Electric or magnetic water conditioning.

Installation, operation and control

8. Check that water softeners will be installed near the incoming supply pipe and where drain access will be available.

9. Check that where an ion exchange water softener is to be installed this will take place downstream of the supply to drinking water points or other equipment or processes which do not require softened water.

10. For water softeners, check that a single check-valve will be installed in dwellings to protect the water supply from backflow. For buildings other than dwellings, the appropriate backflow protection should be provided in accordance with the appropriate fluid category as stated in the *Water Supply (Water Fittings) Regulations 1999* or the *Water Bylaws 2000, Scotland*.

11. Provide a sampling point or tap on the softened water supply from the water softener.

Access and maintenance

12. Provide pipework to bypass the method of water treatment for use in the event of a failure or during maintenance.

13. Provide sufficient space for access for maintenance.

14. Consider the storage and handling of salts.

Economics

15. Consider the likely future cost implication of no water treatment, such as excessive scale build-up resulting in early replacement of equipment and systems and increased operational costs.

16. Consider whole life costs of alternative options.

24 SANITARY ACCOMMODATION REQUIREMENTS

Project title .... **Project No**. .... **Design stage** ....

Engineer .... **Revision No** .... **Date** ....

Checked by .... **Approved by** .... **Date** ....

Design inputs

- Building type and use

- Number of occupants, gender mix, and special needs

- Available water pressure

✓ **Notes / Design file cross-reference**

☐

☐

☐

Design outputs

- Number and location of sanitary fittings

- Specified requirements for sanitary fittings

✓ **Notes / Design file cross-reference**

☐

☐

Key design checks

- Check that the requirements of *Approved Document G1 – Sanitary Conveniences and Washing Facilities* are met

- Check that the requirements of *BS 6465-1* and *BS 6465-2* are followed

- Check that the requirements of *Approved Document F – Ventilation* are met

- Check that the requirements of *Approved Document M – Access to and Use of Buildings* and *BS 8300* are met

- Check that materials and components meet the requirements of the intended building use, design life and maintenance strategy

✓ **Notes / Design file cross-reference**

☐

☐

☐

☐

☐

Project specific checks and notes

✓ **Notes / Design file cross-reference**

☐

☐

☐

24 SANITARY ACCOMMODATION REQUIREMENTS

Design inputs

- Building type and use
- Number of occupants, gender mix, and special needs
- Available water pressure

Design information

- Intended location of sanitary fittings
- Available space for cisterns, valves and pipework

Design outputs

- Number and location of sanitary fittings
- Specified requirements for sanitary fittings

See also: Water Conservation, Cold Water Storage and Distribution, Hot Water Storage and Distribution, Legionnaires' Disease – Cold Water Services, Legionnaires' Disease – Hot Water Services

Key design checks

- Check that the requirements of *Approved Document G1 – Sanitary Conveniences and Washing Facilities* are met
- Check that the requirements of *BS 6465-1* and *BS 6465-2* are followed
- Check that the requirements of *Approved Document F – Ventilation* are met
- Check that the requirements of *Approved Document M – Access to and use of Buildings* and *BS 8300* are met
- Check that materials and components meet the requirements of the intended building use, design life and maintenance strategy

DESIGN WATCHPOINTS

Sizing and selection

1. Check that the provision of sanitary appliances and their location is determined through consultation with the design team at an early stage.
2. Check that WCs or urinals are separated by a door from a room or space where food is prepared or washing up is done. Check that a lobby is included between the room and toilet in the case of a food business.
3. Check whether appliances can be grouped in order to provide economies in pipework.
4. Check that the layout of appliances allows adequate circulation of people and disabled people, where appropriate.
5. Check that hand washing and drying appliances are located between WCs and/or urinals, and the exit, and positioned to prevent congestion.
6. Check that sufficient pressure or flow rate is available when considering direct flush toilets.
7. Check that the selection and siting of items such as toilet paper holders, soap dispensers, shelves, towel cabinets, hand-dryers and disposal bins are considered at the design stage.
8. Check compatibility of all sanitary-ware components, such as cisterns, seats with WC pans and taps with basins.
9. Check that the components selected meet relevant British and European Standards. Confirm with specific clauses to ensure clarity, especially where standards refer to more than one class of product.

Installation, operation and control

10. Check that all appliances, pipework and controls are arranged so as not to obstruct users, and to facilitate cleaning, maintenance and repair.
11. Check that pipework and fittings are enclosed to deter vandalism and accidental damage.
12. Consider the use of non hand-operated taps for basins as they can lead to a reduction in cross infection.
13. Consider the use of spray mixer taps as they can reduce water consumption and result in economies in pipework and energy consumption. Note that in some hard water areas, spray nozzles can rapidly become blocked with lime scale and will involve additional maintenance costs.
14. Consider appliances of robust construction where it is likely that they will be subjected to heavy physical use.
15. Check that WCs, urinals, or washbasins have a surface which is smooth and non-absorbent and capable of being easily cleaned. Consider using anti bacterial surfaces offered by some manufacturers.

16. Check that any flushing apparatus should be capable of cleansing the receptacle effectively. Check that no part of the receptacle is connected to any pipe other than a flush pipe or discharge pipe.
17. Check that all washbasins provided in or adjacent to sanitary accommodation containing a WC or urinal has a supply of hot and cold water.
18. Check that the flushing apparatus of WCs discharges through a trap and discharge pipe into a discharge stack or drain.
19. Check that urinals discharge through a grating, a trap and a branch pipe to a discharge stack or a drain.
20. Check that sanitary appliances, such as WCs and cisterns are ordered as a suite to ensure compatibility.
21. Check that the component parts of the suites are identifiable at all times including delivery, storage and handling on site.

Access and maintenance

22. Select and install appliances correctly to allow subsequent disconnection for maintenance or replacement. Check that appliances are fitted with service valves in accordance with *BS 6675*.
23. Consider the use of wall hung or concealed outlet WC pans as they reduce cleaning work.
24. Provide adequate space around taps to enable ease of use, maintenance and cleaning.
25. Provide a building logbook listing components, manufacturer contact details, expected maintenance regime and frequencies.

Economics

26. Perform a lifecycle cost assessment to ascertain best value based on the expected use, design life of the building and materials in the context of maintenance and replacement periods and consequences of lack of service.
27. Check that dual-flush cisterns default to full flush and display clear instructions on how to operate.
28. Consider the use of water saving devices (see Water Conservation).

25 DRAINAGE SYSTEMS – ABOVE GROUND FOUL DRAINAGE

Project title .... **Project No**... **Design stage**..................

Engineer .... **Revision No**... **Date**...............................

Checked by .... **Approved by**....................................... **Date**...............................

Design inputs

- The number and location of sanitary appliances (consider the likely increase in the use of low-volume flush appliances)

- Height (number of storeys) of building

- Chemical and hazardous waste, and the corrosive nature and temperature of discharges

Notes / Design file cross-reference

Design outputs

- Design of branch discharge pipes, such as pipe size, pipe length, gradient of fall, radius of sweeps, and number of appliances connected

- Design of vertical discharge pipes including stack size, connection of branch discharge pipes, and the radius of bend at the foot of the stack

- Design of ventilation pipes and terminations

- Choice of materials

- Position of drain points for stack connections

Notes / Design file cross-reference

Key design checks

- Design in accordance with *Approved Document H – Drainage and Waste Disposal*

- Design in accordance with *BS EN 12056 – Gravity drainage systems inside buildings*

- Design in accordance with *BS EN 12109 – Vacuum drainage systems inside buildings*

Notes / Design file cross-reference

Project specific checks and notes

Notes / Design file cross-reference

© BSRIA BG2/2006

25 DRAINAGE SYSTEMS – ABOVE GROUND FOUL DRAINAGE

Design inputs

- The number and location of sanitary appliances (consider the likely increase in the use of low-volume flush appliances)
- Height (number of storeys) of building
- Chemical and hazardous waste, and the corrosive nature and temperature of discharges

Design information

- Building type and use
- Occupancy patterns
- Risk of vandalism
- Acoustic requirement
- Fire prevention requirements
- Pipe material and fittings options
- Appliance material options
- Location of pipework – internal or external, exposed or concealed
- Location of gas, water supply, electrical power supply, and other services
- Requirement for grease traps or other types of interceptor traps

Design outputs

- Design of branch discharge pipes, such as pipe size, pipe length, gradient of fall, radius of sweeps, and number of appliances connected
- Design of vertical discharge pipes including stack size, connection of branch discharge pipes, and the radius of bend at the foot of the stack
- Design of ventilation pipes and terminations
- Choice of materials
- Position of drain points for stack connections

Key design checks

- Design in accordance with *Approved Document H – Drainage and Waste Disposal*
- Design in accordance with *BS EN 12056 – Gravity drainage systems inside buildings*
- Design in accordance with *BS EN 12109 – Vacuum drainage systems inside buildings*

See also: Sanitary Accommodation Requirements, Commercial Kitchen Drainage

DESIGN WATCHPOINTS

Sizing and selection

1. Check that the drainage system is designed and installed so that there is adequate hydraulic capacity.
2. Check that the drainage system is water tight and gas tight against operational pressures. Check that vapours and foul air will not be released into the building.
3. Check that provision is made to avoid flooding into the building if there is a risk of flooding from the external drainage system. Follow the requirements of BS EN 12056-4.
4. Check that waste water collected or stored below flood level is discharged into the drainage system via an automatic waste water lifting plant. Follow the requirements of BS EN 12056-4.
5. Check that the risk of blockage under normal conditions is minimised and that the pipework is designed to be self-cleansing through correct pipe sizing and layout.
6. Check that the design will avoid cross-flow between sanitary appliances.
7. Check that drainage is provided for all relevant water supply points inside the building.
8. Check that all appliances connected to the drainage system are installed with a trap. Check that traps on infrequently-used appliances and gullies are protected against the drying out of the water seal.
9. Consider the option of self-sealing waste valves (waterless traps) for condensate drains.
10. Check for each appliance that the minimum trap seal depth, maximum length of pipe from trap outlet to stack, pipe gradient; maximum number of bends, and maximum drop comply with BS EN 12056-2.
11. Check that the capacity of drains is calculated using established formula either directly or by means of tables, charts or appropriate software. (The most widely accepted calculation procedure is the Colebrook-White equation.)
12. Check that pipes serving more than one appliance are sized taking into account the probability of simultaneous discharge. (BS EN 12056-2 provides discharge units for a range of appliances.)
13. Check that the design of branch discharge pipes and vertical discharge pipes complies with BS EN 12056-2.

14. Check that the diameter of discharge pipes are not reduced in the direction of flow.
15. Check that air admittance valves (if used) are sized in accordance with BS EN 12056-2. Note that some local authorities restrict the use of air admittance valves (should not be used where sewers are susceptible to surcharging).
16. Where pipes pass through walls, floors or ceilings subject to fire resistance requirements check that the requirements of Approved Document B – Fire Safety are met.
17. Check that ventilation stacks only serve the drainage systems.
18. Consider the most appropriate pipe material, such as plastics (PVC-u, PP, ABS, and HDPE), cast iron, and stainless steel.
19. Check that the top of open stacks terminate outside the building structure and are positioned such that odours and vapours will not enter the building.
20. Consider the likely noise output from drainage pipes passing through occupied areas. Consider the need for boxing in and/or double-skin pipes. Choose materials with good sound attenuation.
21. For vacuum drainage systems check that the system is designed in accordance with BS EN 12109.
22. Provide grease separators for commercial kitchens (see Commercial Kitchen Drainage).
23. Provide acoustic insulation where materials and location requires it, or specify heavier materials with reduced sound transmission properties.
24. Specify large radius bends at changes of direction to prevent reduction of the flow rate.
25. Consider over-sizing the discharge pipes to reduce the propensity to scale up, especially for branches serving urinals.
26. Avoid complicated knuckle bends and sharp offsets and 92·5° unswept junctions.
27. Check for radioactive discharge from hospitals and laboratories and consider fitting an alarm probe into the drainage system for radioactive discharges.

25 DRAINAGE SYSTEMS – ABOVE GROUND FOUL DRAINAGE

DESIGN WATCHPOINTS

Installation, operation and control

28. Check that the system is designed and built so that it can resist the loading likely to act on it during the installation and building works.

29. Consider the effect of thermal movement and follow the pipe manufacturers instructions.

30. Check that pipes with joints allowing longitudinal movement are fixed and/or supported so that joints cannot become unintentionally disconnected.

31. Check that pipework fixing is secure and stable, and will not cause damage to pipework or parts of the building.

32. Check that the pipework is suitably supported.

33. Check that other services are not attached to the pipework.

34. Check that the external surfaces of pipes do not come into contact with materials likely to attack them, for example from electrolytic or chemical action.

35. Check that pipes installed in floors or walls are suitably protected and that the effects of expansion or shrinkage of the surrounding material is considered.

36. Check that purpose-made fittings are specified for the connection of pipes made of different material and/or sizes.

37. Check that sanitary appliances are connected to the wastewater discharge pipe using manufacturers' recommended fittings.

38. Check that suitable pipes and fitting materials are selected according to the likely waste matter and temperature of waste being discharged to the drainage system, such as high temperature waste from autoclaves, and chemical material from laboratories.

39. Consider health and safety implications particularly with long, heavy pipes and chemical solvents. Check that *COSHH Regulations* are in place.

40. Check that guidance is included in the operation and maintenance manual concerning maintenance activities and frequencies.

Access and maintenance

41. Check the provision of adequate access to enable testing, inspection and maintenance. Ensure that access is provided for all traps, discharge pipes and stacks to allow clearance of blockages. Check that access is provided at each change of direction to allow rodding to take place.

42. Provide operation and maintenance information for the building owner or occupier.

43. Consider the maintenance costs of joints, such as replacing seals, and caulking.

Economics

44. Consider capital costs and through-life costs when making specifying decisions about pipe material.

45. Consider costs and system choice on the risk and consequences of blockages and leaks.

46. Consider that installation costs may be reduced by specifying push-fit systems.

47. Consider that rigid lightweight systems may need fewer fixings and have reduced installation costs.

48. Consider the costs associated with providing fire insulation or acoustic insulation. This should be considered when making pipework material choices.

© BSRIA BG2/2006

26 FOUL WATER – BELOW GROUND DRAINAGE SYSTEMS

Project title .... **Project No**. .... **Design stage** ....

Engineer .... **Revision No** .... **Date** ....

Checked by .... **Approved by** .... **Date** ....

Design inputs

Notes / Design file cross-reference

- Distance between development and public sewer (if available) and invert levels at point of connection ❑
- Building type and use ❑
- Number of building occupants and occupancy patterns ❑
- Number and type of sanitary fittings ❑

Design outputs

Notes / Design file cross-reference

- Pipe size, gradient and layout ❑
- Pumping and anti-flooding requirements ❑

Key design checks

Notes / Design file cross-reference

- Check that the requirements of *Approved Document H1 – Foul Water Drainage* are complied with ❑
- Note that the requirement of *H1* can also be met by following Parts 3,4 and 6 of *BS EN 752* together with *BS EN 1610*, *BS EN 1295* and *BS EN 12056-2* ❑
- Check that the drains will have enough capacity to carry the design flow ❑
- Consider consequences of surcharging ❑

Project specific checks and notes

Notes / Design file cross-reference

❑

❑

❑

© BSRIA BG2/2006

26 FOUL WATER BELOW GROUND DRAINAGE SYSTEMS

Design inputs

- Distance between development and public sewer (if available) and invert levels at point of connection
- Building type and use
- Number of building occupants and occupancy patterns
- Number and type of sanitary fittings

Design information

- Details of agreement with the sewerage undertaker regarding connection to the public sewer, such as adoption on completion or sewer requisition, permissible flow rates, and trade waste discharges
- Requirement for any wastewater treatment system
- Extent and possible frequency of potential surcharging
- Requirement for special measures for the control of rodents
- CCTV survey of existing drains (if required)
- Level of sewer or drain connection point
- External ground levels and internal ground floor levels

Design outputs

- Pipe size, gradient and layout
- Pumping and anti-flooding requirements

Key design checks

- Check that the requirements of *Approved Document H1 – Foul Water Drainage* are complied with
- Note that the requirement of *H1* can also be met by following Parts 3,4 and 6 of *BS EN 752* together with *BS EN 1610*, *BS EN 1295* and *BS EN 12056-2*
- Check that the drains will have enough capacity to carry the design flow
- Consider consequences of surcharging

See also: Local Authority Requirements and Discharge Consents, Foul Water Below Ground Drainage System Sizing, Drainage Systems – Above Ground Foul Drainage, Commercial Kitchen Drainage, Sustainable Urban Drainage Systems

DESIGN WATCHPOINTS

Sizing and selection

1. Determine the design approach for dealing with surcharging of drains. Consider pumping installations, anti-flooding valves, or the use of a gully outside the building.
2. Check that any sanitary fittings or outlets which are not more than 1 m above the local authority's sewer surcharge level are not connected directly into a sewer.
3. For pumping installations, choose between an inside or outside installation. For inside pumping installations, check for compliance with BS EN 12050 and BS EN 12056-4. For outside pumping installations check for compliance with BS EN 752-6.
4. Check that anti-flooding valves are suitable for foul water, comply with BS EN 13564, are of the double valve type, and have a manual closure device.
5. Check that gullies are at least 75 mm below floor level and positioned so that flooding from them will not damage any buildings.
6. Check that all drainage unaffected by surcharge will bypass any protective measures and discharge by gravity.
7. Check that appropriate measures will be taken to control rodents, such as sealed drainage, interception trap stoppers, rodent barriers, metal cages on ventilator stack terminals, and covers and gratings that can be fixed in position.
8. Check that drains will have enough capacity to carry the design flow. Check that the recommendations provided in *Approved Document H1* and BS EN 12056 are followed.
9. Carry out a risk assessment of the building, its use and its ground conditions in order to select the most suitable material for the drainage pipework. Consider contaminated ground, ground movement, and the presence of chemicals.
10. If the drainage is to be adopted by the local authority, check that is has been designed in accordance with latest edition of *Sewers for adoption*.
11. Check suitable termination for drain vents.
12. Check co-ordination of the drainage system with the building substructure.
13. Check the co-ordination of the drainage system with other external services.
14. Check that suitable bedding systems will be specified for the pipe material, depth, ground conditions and expected surface loads if applicable.

Installation, operation and control

15. Check that where an anti-flooding valve is to be installed, a notice is provided indicating that the system should be drained through the valve, and also indicates the location of any manual override.
16. Check that the layout of the drainage system is kept as simple as possible. Minimise changes of direction and gradient.
17. Check that the connection of drains is accomplished with easy sweeps in the direction of flow. Check that connections will be made using prefabricated components.
18. Check that repair couplings will be used when connecting to existing drains or sewers. Check that the junction will be carefully packed to avoid differential settlement with adjacent pipes.
19. Check that the drainage system will be properly ventilated.
20. Check that pipes will be laid to even gradients with access points provided where a change of gradient occurs.
21. Check that pipes will be laid in straight lines where practicable. Check that any bends will have a large a radius as is practicable. Check that bends will be limited to positions in, or close to, inspection chambers or manholes, and to the foot of discharge and ventilation stacks.
22. Check that adequate measures will be taken to provide protection from settlement.
23. Check that a water tightness test will be performed after completion (either an air test or water test).
24. Check for radioactive discharge from hospitals and laboratory equipment. Consider fitting a radioactive discharge probe into the drainage system.

Access and maintenance

25. Provide adequate access for cleaning.
26. Check that the requirements of *Approved Document H1* are met with regard to the minimum dimensions for access fittings and inspection chambers, minimum dimensions for manholes, and maximum spacing of access points.

Economics

27. Weigh up cost options of pipe material and bedding requirements for expected loadings.

27 COMMERCIAL KITCHEN DRAINAGE

Project title .... **Project No** .... **Design stage** ....

Engineer .... **Revision No** .... **Date** ....

Checked by .... **Approved by** .... **Date** ....

Design inputs

Notes / Design file cross-reference

- Specification of sinks, dishwasher and waste disposal units ☐
- Highest number of meals served daily (number of covers) ☐
- Waste pipe and drain diameters ☐
- Hours of kitchen use ☐

Design outputs

Notes / Design file cross-reference

- Size and type of grease separators ☐
- Requirements for dosing of grease traps ☐
- Type of drainage pipework ☐
- Arrangement for branch discharge pipes ☐
- Temperature of discharges and flow rates from equipment ☐
- Requirements for drainage channels for Bratt Pan discharges ☐
- Suitable pipe materials depending on temperature ☐

Key design checks

Notes / Design file cross-reference

- For compliance with *Approved Document H1*, check that a grease separator is installed as necessary or grease treatment provided (enzyme dosing could be preferable to interceptors) ☐
- Check that the grease separator is correctly sized and installed ☐
- Check the drainage requirements for specific kitchen appliances ☐

Project specific checks and notes

Notes / Design file cross-reference

☐
☐
☐

27 COMMERCIAL KITCHEN DRAINAGE

Design inputs

- Specification of sinks, dishwasher and waste disposal units
- Highest number of meals served daily (number of covers)
- Waste pipe and drain diameters
- Hours of kitchen use

Design information

- History of blockages and drainage problems for existing sites
- Application of the kitchen
- Details of drain runs and manholes

See also: Local Authority Requirements and Discharge Consents, Drainage Systems – Above Ground Foul Drainage, Foul Water Below Ground Drainage Systems

Design outputs

- Size and type of grease separators
- Requirements for dosing of grease traps
- Type of drainage pipework
- Arrangement for branch discharge pipes
- Temperature of discharges and flow rates from equipment
- Requirements for drainage channels for Bratt Pan discharges
- Suitable pipe materials depending on temperature

Key design checks

- For compliance with *Approved Document H1* check that a grease separator is installed as necessary or grease treatment provided (enzyme dosing could be preferable to interceptors)
- Check that the grease separator is correctly sized and installed
- Check the drainage requirements for specific kitchen appliances

DESIGN WATCHPOINTS

Sizing and selection

1. Check that kitchen drainage pipework is robust enough to receive high temperature discharges.
2. Check that kitchen drainage systems will not be closely linked to other parts of the building. Check that separate drainage stacks are provided where kitchens are located other than on the ground floor. This is advisable in order to avoid backflow problems.
3. Check that a grease separator is provided in order to comply with *Approved Document H1 – Foul Water Drainage*.
4. Check that the grease separator complies with *BS EN 1825-1* and is designed and installed in accordance with *BS EN 1825-2*.
5. Check that the sizing of the grease separator is based on: maximum flow rate of wastewater, maximum temperature of the wastewater, density of grease/oils to be separated, and the influence of cleansing and rinsing agents.
6. Consider the use of dosed chemical injection.
7. Consider the use of retention units that heat the wastewater to allow the automatic skimming and removal of grease.

Installation, operation and control

8. Check that the requirements of *BS EN 12056-2* are followed.
9. Check that only kitchen appliances generating grease are connected to the grease separator, as other wastes, such as vegetable matter, will interfere with the working of the unit.
10. Check that the grease separator will be installed close to the sources of waste water. Where this is not possible and/or the pipe(s) will be installed in cool areas, consider the requirement for thermally insulating the pipe(s).
11. Consider the requirement for trace heating of pipes in areas prone to frost. Where trace heating is required, check that the heating is controlled by a time clock in order to avoid unnecessary heating.
12. Check that the separator will be installed such that it will be protected from frost.
13. Check that, where possible, grease separators are installed externally. Avoid installations within kitchens. Check that they are not installed in food storage preparation areas. Check that the separator will not be sited close to openable windows and air intakes in order to prevent potential odour problems and check that it is installed within the required maximum distance of the equipment to which it is connected.

14. For below ground grease separators consider whether heavy-duty covers are required.
15. Check that pipes upstream of the separator will have a minimum gradient of 2% in order to prevent the accumulation of grease.
16. Check that discharge points will have traps with sediment buckets that can be removed for cleaning. Check that upstream and downstream pipes connected to grease separators will be adequately ventilated.
17. Where the kitchen is to be pumped, check that either a grease trap or chemical dosing feed is installed to prevent grease coagulation.
18. Avoid the use of floor channels, open gullies and gratings in kitchens and associated areas due to their unhygienic nature.
19. Check that sinks and washing up machines are individually trapped and directly connected to the drainage system.
20. Check that vegetable-paring machines will be fitted with a waste dilution unit that is trapped and directly connected to the drainage system.
21. Check application of increased gradients from waste disposal units and try to ensure that other fittings upstream provide additional water for flushing through.
22. Check that pipes from kitchen appliances containing heavy concentrations of solid matter will be connected as close as possible to the main drain or discharge stack. Avoid connections to long runs of horizontal pipes.
23. Avoid internal manholes if possible.

Access and maintenance

24. Check that grease separators will be installed to allow easy access for removal of grease and for maintenance and cleaning.
25. Consider the likely emptying frequency for the grease separator. If this is excessive consider the use of automated systems (automatic skimming of the grease into a container for removal).
26. Consider maintenance regimes for enzyme-dosing systems.

Economics

27. Perform a cost assessment of pipe and grease separator options for expected level or use and the maintenance regimes.

28   SURFACE WATER – BELOW GROUND DRAINAGE SYSTEMS

Project title.. **Project No**........................... **Design stage**.................

Engineer... **Revision No**........................ **Date**.............................

Checked by... **Approved by**............................ **Date**................

Design inputs

- Rainfall intensities, durations and return period

- Water catchment area

- Level of local water table

- Distance between the development and the public sewer and invert level

✓ **Notes / Design file cross-reference**

☐

☐

☐

☐

Design outputs

- Size, layout and gradient of required drainage pipework

- Requirement for any water treatment/oil interceptors /separators

✓ **Notes / Design file cross-reference**

☐

☐

Key design checks

- Check that the requirements of *Approved Document H3 – Rainwater Drainage* are met. Note that the requirements of *Approved Document H3* can be met by following the relevant recommendations of BS EN 752-4

- Check that the drains will have enough capacity to carry the design flow

- Consider consequences of surcharging

- Check for compliance with Environment Agency *PPG3*

- Check that rainwater will discharge to one of the following in order of priority: adequate soakaway or some other adequate infiltration system, a water course, a sewer

✓ **Notes / Design file cross-reference**

☐

☐

☐

☐

☐

Project specific checks and notes

✓ **Notes / Design file cross-reference**

☐

☐

☐

28 SURFACE WATER BELOW GROUND DRAINAGE SYSTEMS

Design inputs

- Rainfall intensities, durations and return period
- Water catchment area
- Level of local water table
- Distance between the development and the public sewer and invert level

Design information

- Details of agreement with the sewerage undertaker regarding connection to the public sewer, permissible flow rates, and invert level at the point of proposed connection
- Details of sources of water pollution
- Suitability of surrounding area for infiltration drainage systems
- Requirement for a water treatment system
- Extent and possible frequency of potential surcharging
- Level of sewer or drain connection point
- External ground levels and site topography
- Run-off coefficient (impermeability factor) of external surfaces

See also: Local Authority Requirements and Discharge Consents, Sustainable Urban Drainage Systems, Reclaimed Water Systems– General, Reclaimed Water Systems – Greywater, Reclaimed Water Systems– Rainwater

Design outputs

- Size, layout and gradient of required drainage pipework
- Requirement for any water treatment, oil interceptors and separators

Key design checks

- Check that the requirements of *Approved Document H3 – Rainwater Drainage* are met. Note that the requirements of *Approved Document H3* can be met by following the relevant recommendations of *BS EN 752-4*
- Check that the drains will have enough capacity to carry the design flow
- Consider consequences of surcharging
- Check for compliance with Environment Agency *PPG3*
- Check that rainwater will discharge to one of the following in order of priority: adequate soakaway or some other adequate infiltration system, a water course, a sewer

DESIGN WATCHPOINTS

Sizing and selection

1. Consider whether gravity connection to sewers is impractical or surcharging of sewers is likely. Consider the use of surface-water lifting equipment.
2. Check whether materials that could act as a source of pollution will be present. If this is the case check that either a separate drainage system will be provided capable of dealing with the polluted effluent, or a separator or treatment system is needed.
3. Check that oil interceptors will be provided for areas where a leakage or spillage of oil is likely, such as in car parks and petrol filling stations. Check that the requirements detailed in *Appendix H3-A of Approved Document H3* are followed.
4. Check whether a combined sewer arrangement is appropriate. Where this is the case, check that traps on all inlets to the combined sewer will be installed.
5. Consider whether infiltration drainage systems may be used, such as soakaways, swales, infiltration basins and filter drains.
6. Check that infiltration drainage systems will not be built:
   - Within 5 m of a building or road or in areas of unstable land.
   - Where the water table would reach the bottom of the system at any time of the year.
   - Contamination in the run-off could pollute the groundwater.
   - Where insufficient drainage exists (soil infiltration rate).
7. For soakaways check that:
   - The design guidance in *National Annex NG* of *BS EN 752-4* is followed.
   - Ground permeability test figures are obtained to determine whether the ground is suitable. *BRE Digest 365* includes a test methodology for the measurement of soil infiltration rates.
   - Adequate provision is made for inspection and maintenance.
   - A suitable oil interceptor is provided (if required) if the run-off water will come from a paved surface.
8. For drainage from paved areas consider the use of pervious paving and/or or the use of free-draining surfaces.
9. For drainage systems from impervious paving, check that they are designed in accordance with *National Annex NE* of *BS EN 752-4*.
10. Carry out a risk assessment of the building, its use and ground conditions in order to select the most suitable material for the drainage pipework, such as contaminated ground, ground movement, and the presence of chemicals.
11. If the drainage system is to be adopted by the local authority, check that it has been designed in accordance with the latest edition of *Sewers for Adoption*.

12. Check that a suitable bedding system is specified for the pipe material, depth and consider expected surface loads if applicable.

Installation, operation and control

13. Check that the layout of the drainage system is kept as simple as possible. Minimise changes of direction and gradient.
14. Check that connection of drains is accomplished with easy sweeps in the direction of flow. Check that connections will be made using prefabricated components.
15. Check that repair couplings will be used when connecting existing drains or sewers. Check that the junction will be carefully packed to avoid differential settlement with adjacent pipes.
16. Check that the drainage system will be properly ventilated.
17. Check that pipes will be laid to even gradients with access points provided where a change of gradient occurs.
18. Check that pipes will be laid in straight lines where practicable. Check that any bends will have a large a radius as practicable. Check that bends will be limited to positions in or close to inspection chambers of manholes and to the foot of discharge and ventilation stacks.
19. Check that the correct choice of bedding and backfilling is made (this will depend on the type of pipes to be laid and ground conditions).
20. Check that a water tightness test will be performed after completion (either an air test or water test).

Access and maintenance

21. Provide adequate access for cleaning.
22. Check that the requirements of *Approved Document H1* are followed with respect to minimum dimensions for access fittings and inspection chambers, minimum dimensions for manholes, and maximum spacing of access points.
23. Check that provision is made for the cleaning and maintenance of interceptors.

Economics

24. Weigh up the costs of different pipe materials, and bedding requirements for expected loadings.
25. Consider carrying out a whole life costing assessment for alternative surface water drainage systems, including soakaway and recycling options.

29 ROOF DRAINAGE

Project title.. **Project No**.. **Design stage**.................

Engineer.. **Revision No**.. **Date**...............................

Checked by.. **Approved by**...................................... **Date**...............................

Design inputs

✓ **Notes / Design file cross-reference**

- Roof dimensions ❑

- Return period ❑

- Design rainfall intensity and duration ❑

- Life expectancy of the building ❑

- Decide gravity or siphonic systems ❑

Design outputs

✓ **Notes / Design file cross-reference**

- Required gutter capacity and outlet size ❑

- Required rainwater pipe sizes ❑

Key design checks

✓ **Notes / Design file cross-reference**

- Design in accordance with *Approved Document H – Drainage and Waste Disposal* ❑

- Design in accordance with *BS EN 12056-3* ❑

Project specific checks and notes

✓ **Notes / Design file cross-reference**

❑

❑

❑

29 ROOF DRAINAGE

Design inputs

- Roof dimensions
- Return period
- Design rainfall intensity and duration
- Life expectancy of the building
- Decide gravity or siphonic systems

Design information

- Geographical location
- Building type and location
- Type of roof drainage, such as a flat roof with outlets or pitched roof with parapet and eaves gutter
- Architects allowance regarding downpipes (consultation with the architect should take place at an early stage in the design)
- Type of outfall drainage available in order of priority: soakaway, watercourse, and sewer

Design outputs

- Required gutter capacity and outlet size
- Required rainwater pipe sizes

Key design checks

- Design in accordance with *Approved Document H – Drainage and Waste Disposal*
- Design in accordance with *BS EN 12056-3*

See Also: Sustainable Urban Drainage Systems

DESIGN WATCHPOINTS

Sizing and selection

1. Check that run-off calculations have been performed (including any run-off from vertical surfaces).
2. Check that an appropriate return period has been selected, with due regard to the life of the building and seriousness of the consequences of any flooding to the building. Anticipate the lifespan of the building when selecting a return period. Consult and agree with the client the selected return period.
3. Check that the effective catchment area has been calculated.
4. Check that the design capacity of gutters has been determined. Check the outlet size.
5. Check that the capacity of rainwater pipes is adequate and that the design flow rates through the outlets can be achieved.
6. For siphonic systems check that the requirements of *BS EN 12056-3* (section 6.2) have been met and that the below ground drainage system will be sized to receive concentrated flow. Check that the system supplier has been consulted.
7. Check that the design of the roof drainage system takes into account construction tolerances and settlement so as to avoid backfalls and ponding.
8. Check that the gradient of eaves gutters are not so steep that the gutters drop below the level of the roof to such an extent that water discharging from the roof will pass over the edge of the gutter.
9. For flat roofs with parapets, check that at least two outlets (or one outlet plus an emergency overflow) are provided for each roof area. Consider the importance of emergency overflow requirements.
10. Check that the reduction in outlet capacity due to strainers installed in outlets has been taken into account.
11. Check that overflows or emergency outlets are provided on flat roofs with parapets and in non-eaves gutters.
12. For horizontal and near horizontal pipelines, check that increases in size are specified such that the soffit is continuous in order to prevent air from being trapped (for example, use eccentric coupling, to achieve level soffit).
13. Check that internal rainwater pipes will be able to withstand the head of water likely to occur in the event of a blockage.
14. Check that pipework does not reduce in diameter in the direction of flow (except for siphonic systems).
15. Check that pipe shoes are specified where there is no alternative to a rainwater pipe discharging on to a lower roof or paved area. The covering of the roof should be reinforced at the point where the pipe shoe discharges.
16. Check for the inclusion of leaf guards.
17. Check for compatibility between component parts to ensure no bimetallic corrosion. Check that gutter material is compatible with the roof covering material.

Installation, operation and control

18. Check that nominally level gutters will be laid with a gradient between one millimetre per metre and three millimetres per metre where practical.
19. Check that a watertight seal is specified for pipes that pass through the external walls of the building.
20. Check that where a rainwater pipe will discharge into a gully, it will terminate below the gully grating but above the seal.
21. Check that pipework will be insulated if condensation is likely to present a problem.
22. Consideration should be given to frost protection and snow guards. The use of electrical trace heating may be appropriate in vulnerable areas.
23. Assess the likely noise output from rainwater pipes passing through occupied spaces. Consider the need for boxing in and/or double skin pipes – choose materials with low dB rating. Consider the need for acoustic insulation.

Access and maintenance

24. Check that rainwater pipes are not encased in structural elements of buildings. Where they are installed in ducts or casings, check that they will be accessible for inspection, maintenance, repair and replacement.
25. Provide access for cleaning and inspection above the foot of rainwater stacks and at changes in direction where there is a risk of blockage.
26. Where applicable, check that access points will not be sited in habitable rooms.
27. Check that a maintenance logbook will be prepared that emphasises the importance of clearing gutters annually and after storms, particularly if the building's in an area with trees.

Economics

28. Carry out a life-cycle cost assessment to ascertain best value based on the design life of the building and materials used for the drainage system, maintenance and replacement periods.
29. Consider a trade-off between seamless gutters and those with seals (seals require replacement and may leak).

© BSRIA BG2/2006

30 SUSTAINABLE URBAN DRAINAGE SYSTEMS

Project title... **Project No**.. **Design stage**..................

Engineer.. **Revision No**.................................... **Date**..............................

Checked by.. **Approved by**................................. **Date**..............................

Design inputs

- Rainfall data (meet Environment Agency requirements)
- Quantity and discharge design criteria
- Hydrology of catchment
- Level of local water table

✓ **Notes / Design file cross-reference**

☐
☐
☐

Design outputs

- Run-off
- Design treatment volume
- Type, location and size of drainage devices
- Flow rates for discharge off-site
- Material options which meet the expected service life of the system

✓ **Notes / Design file cross-reference**

☐
☐
☐
☐
☐

Key design checks

- Determine the risk of sensitive groundwater contamination
- Take steps to lower peak flows to watercourses or sewers in order to replicate natural land drainage and reduce flood risk
- Replicate natural drainage patterns so that changes to base flows are minimal
- Where possible, provide treatment of run-off to improve its water quality
- Check that materials and components are suitable for the expected system life

✓ **Notes / Design file cross-reference**

☐
☐
☐
☐
☐

Project specific checks and notes

✓ **Notes / Design file cross-reference**

☐
☐
☐

30 SUSTAINABLE URBAN DRAINAGE SYSTEMS

Design inputs

- Rainfall data (meet Environment Agency requirements)
- Quantity and discharge design criteria
- Hydrology of catchment
- Level of local water table

Design information

- Former land use and topography
- Quantity and discharge design criteria
- Details of receiving sewer, watercourse or aquifer
- Soil type and infiltration potential
- Presence of environmentally sensitive area, groundwater protection zones
- Development type and land use
- Sub-catchment types within the development
- Porosity of ground (based on percolation tests)
- Expected service life of the system
- Legislative responsibilities concerning adoption

See also: Future Needs

Design outputs

- Run-off
- Design treatment volume
- Type, location and size of drainage devices
- Flow rates for discharge off-site
- Material options which meet the expected service life of the system

Key design checks

- Determine the risk of sensitive groundwater contamination
- Take steps to lower peak flows to watercourses or sewers in order to replicate natural land drainage and reduce flood risk
- Replicate natural drainage patterns so that changes to base flows are minimal
- Where possible, provide treatment of run-off to improve its water quality
- Check that materials and components are suitable for the expected system life

DESIGN WATCHPOINTS

Sizing and selection

1. Determine design flood frequencies.
2. Consider steps to attenuate run-off. Minimise the amount of paved or compacted surfaces. Consider the use of gravelled surfaces as an alternative to tarmac in parking areas.
3. Consider whether hard paving and roofed areas can be drained onto unpaved areas. Aim to return run-off to the natural drainage system as soon as possible.
4. As a design objective, check if the run-off hydrograph will be similar before and after development. (The time of concentration and baseflow resulting from the development should be broadly similar to those from the undeveloped site.)
5. Determine baseflows to ensure watercourses and ponds do not dry out.
6. Check that the method to estimate the catchment response has been agreed. (Data for flow estimation methods can be obtained from sewerage undertakers, local authorities and the Environment Agency.)
7. Check that the amount of run-off has been estimated.
8. Be aware that the hydraulic design of sustainable urban drainage systems (SUDS) is subjected to a greater level of uncertainty than conventional pipe systems. Calculations are subject to individual judgement and some sensitivity analysis may be necessary for critical designs.
9. Consider and select suitable methods to deal with run-off rates. Potential options include:
   - permeable surfaces
   - filter strips
   - swales
   - soakaways and infiltration trenches
   - filter drains
   - infiltration basins
   - detention basins
   - retention ponds
   - wetlands.
10. Determine the level of pollution risk and the sensitivity of the receiving water environment if infiltration is to be adopted. Check that soil infiltration tests have been performed.
11. Consider the use of canopies over areas of potentially high contamination as this removes the risk of surface water becoming polluted.
12. Consider the use of silt traps and downpipe filters which will help to treat run-off before it reaches the drainage system.
13. Check that infiltration is not used in areas where contamination of sensitive groundwater could occur (see the Environment Agency's protection zone maps).

14. Be aware that construction activity may compact soils and reduce infiltration.
15. Determine the number and type of treatment strategies required.
16. Consider the pollution prevention requirements associated with areas such as fuel tanks and rubbish skips.
17. Determine which areas need to be connected to the foul sewer (subject to the agreement of the sewerage undertaker).
18. Check that the design includes adequate means of capturing and treating polluted run-off following storms. (The amount of treatment necessary will depend on the forecast level of pollution.)
19. For developments on contaminated land, check and demonstrate to the Environment Agency that the proposed drainage system will not cause movement of contaminants.
20. Consider whether run-off can be used to improve facilities for the local community and wildlife.
21. Conduct a safety review to determine which designs are inherently safe for the specific application. Determine whether access to specific areas needs to be restricted or discouraged.

Installation, operation and control

22. Consider whether the construction site will require any additional drainage measures such as:
    - temporary pre-treatment before run-off enters the drainage system
    - infiltration measures or permeable surfaces to protect from silt during construction activity
    - protection for plants until they have become established.

Access and maintenance

23. Consider the maintenance requirements of the intended design.
24. Check that appropriate maintenance procedures will be put in place.
25. Verify who will be responsible for maintaining the system.
26. Check maintenance requirements and frequencies are listed in a logbook.

Economics

27. Availability and cost of land.
28. Perform a whole-life cost assessment of options and ensure best value is struck between capital costs and in use costs, particularly if those constructing the sustainable urban drainage systems (SUDS) will not be responsible for any maintenance.
29. Review costs with the funder before submission to authority.

© BSRIA BG2/2006

31 RECLAIMED WATER SYSTEMS – GENERAL

Project title .... **Project No.** .... **Design stage** ....

Engineer .... **Revision No** .... **Date** ....

Checked by .... **Approved by** .... **Date** ....

Design inputs

☑ **Notes / Design file cross-reference**

- Water demand and use ☐
- Likely available sources and quantity of water for recovery ☐
- Quality and chemical composition of available water ☐

Design outputs

☑ **Notes / Design file cross-reference**

- Size and location of storage tanks ☐
- Size and location of pre-filters, and water treatment plant ☐
- Consideration of the material and quality criteria for the component parts for durability and reliability for a given set of conditions ☐
- Structural requirements for water storage support, particularly if in a roof space. Alternatively, detail relating to the installation of the tank in the ground ☐

Key design checks

☑ **Notes / Design file cross-reference**

- Check that the design complies with the *Water Supply (Water Fittings) Regulations 1999* and the *Water Byelaws 2000, Scotland* ☐
- Check that any connections made to a soakaway, storm-water drain or foul drainage system is undertaken in consultation with the sewerage undertaker and follows the requirements of *Approved Document H – Drainage and Waste Disposal* ☐
- Check that a hazard assessment protocol is followed when a reclaimed water system is to be installed or modified (see WRAS *Information and Guidance Note 9-02-04*) ☐
- Check that reclaimed water systems are not used for drinking, food preparation, cooking or bathing, unless the design, installation, operation and maintenance (including regular water quality monitoring) complies with potable water standards and regulations (Fluid Category1, *Water Supply (Water Fittings) Regulations 1999*) ☐
- Check that the correct terminology is used: ☐
  - Reclaimed water: water which has been treated so that its quality is suitable for particular specified purposes such as irrigation and toilet flushing
  - Greywater: water originally supplied as wholesome water that has already been used for bathing, washing, laundry or washing dishes

Project specific checks and notes

☑ **Notes / Design file cross-reference**

☐

☐

31   RECLAIMED WATER SYSTEMS – GENERAL

Design inputs

- Water demand and use
- Likely available sources and quantity of water for recovery
- Quality and chemical composition of available water

Design information

- Available space and location for storage tanks
- Available drainage
- Required water treatment and disinfection
- Check acceptability with the water authority

Design outputs

- Size and location of storage tanks
- Size and location of pre-filters, and water treatment plant
- Consideration of the material and quality criteria for the component parts for durability and reliability for a given set of conditions
- Structural requirements for water storage support, particularly if in a roof space. Alternatively, detail relating to the installation of the tank in the ground

See Also: Cold Water Storage and Distribution, Legionnaires' Disease – Cold Water Services, Reclaimed Water Systems – Greywater, Reclaimed Water Systems – Rainwater
Note: Reference must be made to Reclaimed Water Systems – Greywater and Reclaimed Water Systems – Rainwater where relevant

Key design checks

- Check that the design complies with the *Water Supply (Water Fittings) Regulations 1999* and the *Water Byelaws 2000, Scotland*
- Check that any connections made to a soakaway, storm-water drain or foul drainage system is undertaken in consultation with the sewerage undertaker and follows the requirements of *Approved Document H – Drainage and Waste Disposal*
- Check that a hazard assessment protocol is followed when a reclaimed water system is to be installed or modified (see WRAS *Information and Guidance Note 9-02-04*)
- Check that reclaimed water systems are not used for drinking, food preparation, cooking or bathing, unless the design, installation, operation and maintenance (including regular water quality monitoring) complies with potable water standards and regulations (Fluid Category1, *Water Supply (Water Fittings) Regulations 1999*)
- Check that the correct terminology is used:
  - Reclaimed water: water which has been treated so that its quality is suitable for particular specified purposes such as irrigation and toilet flushing
  - Greywater: water originally supplied as wholesome water that has already been used for bathing, washing, laundry or washing dishes

---

DESIGN WATCHPOINTS

Sizing and selection

1. Confirm that components and materials comply with *The Water Fittings Materials Directory* and BS 6920.
2. Check that mains water supplies are not cross-connected with reclaimed water. Follow the WRAS pipework colour coding for the identification of reclaimed-water pipework.
3. Check that ingress of contamination into the collection tank is prevented by a raised cover or sealed lid. (Check that the lid can be secured to prevent unauthorised entry.)
4. Check that tanks are protected from rodents or insects with an appropriate screen or trap and vented to avoid gas build-up.
5. Check that tanks are designed to prevent the ingress of ground water that may be contaminated.
6. When sizing storage tanks, check that an allowance is made for residues that will build up over time.
7. Check that the tank design promotes settlement of solids at the bottom. Check that inlets and draw-off points should be located to avoid disturbing sediment at the bottom of the tank.
8. Check that backflow prevention is provided to avoid storm drains, soakaways, and sewers, backing up into collection tanks.
9. Check that a type AA or AB air gap for the prevention of backflow (in compliance with the *Water Supply Regulations*) is provided where mains top-up to a direct supply system is used.
10. Check that a type AA or AB air gap is provided where a mains top-up to a high-level cistern or an indirect gravity-fed supply system is used.
11. Consider providing the ability to divert the mains water supply without the need for user intervention.
12. Check that copper and galvanised steel pipes are not used due to the acidic nature of rainwater and the high level of salts present in greywater.

13. Check that corrosion-resistant components such as plastic pipe and fittings are specified. If chemical cleaning is to be used, check the likely levels of bromine or chlorine may degrade some plastic and rubber materials used in conventional plumbing.
14. Check that appropriate methods of water treatment and disinfection are provided, this will be a function of the intended use for the water.
15. Consider the use of filtration incorporating self-cleaning and automatic back-washing processes.
16. Consider applying chemical disinfection at the collection tank so that all the stored water is treated.
17. Check that chemical disinfection is not applied before any biological treatment or before membrane filters.
18. Check that the intended system components are compatible with the chemical disinfectants.
19. Check that a fail-safe mechanism is used that diverts to waste untreated water if the supply of disinfectant runs out.
20. Check that the pump is corrosion resistant and is of the correct duty. Provide a means of ensuring that the pump is protected from dry running.
21. Check that the system is designed to minimise the possibility of blockages and residue build up.

Installation, operation and control

22. Contact the local planning and building control authorities before installing external tanks.
23. Check that underground tanks are designed and installed to withstand groundwater, earth and/or backfill pressure, surcharge loads, vehicular loads and flotation.
24. Check that where separate potable and greywater/rainwater cisterns are installed, each is clearly marked to show their intended use.
25. Check that rainwater tanks overflow to a soakaway or storm water drain and not to a foul sewer.

31 RECLAIMED WATER SYSTEMS – GENERAL

DESIGN WATCHPOINTS

Installation, operation and control

26. Check that greywater tanks overflow to the foul drainage system.

27. Check that tanks and associated pipework situated above ground are sufficiently insulated to prevent freezing.

28. Check that the design of the distribution system avoids dead legs or infrequently-used outlets.

29. Include a control system that provides visual alarm indicators for common fault conditions such as pump failure, disinfection failure and filter blockage. Link to a building management system if appropriate.

30. Check that if the system fails to operate it will default to potable mains water back-up supply.

31. Check that any equipment or apparatus supplied with recycled water will carry a warning label.

32. Check that access points will be provided for maintenance and the clearing of blockages.

33. Check that adequate ventilation will be provided to prevent the possibility of foul air accumulating in the installation or drainage system.

34. Check that reclaimed water systems used for irrigation will not result in the contamination of any watercourses and aquifers.

Access and maintenance

35. Check that tanks are accessible for periodic internal cleaning and the maintenance of system components such as valves, pumps and sensors. Check that a close fitting removable cover is specified.

36. Check that the system is designed to be taken out of use to allow tanks to be emptied and prevented from refilling or supplying water to the point of use.

37. Check that suitable installation, operation and maintenance manuals are provided. Check that instructions are included for the safe disposal of treatment chemicals or waste residues.

38. Specify that systems are indelibly labelled with the model number and manufacturer's name and contact details in case the original documentation is lost.

39. Consider the risk of personnel being trapped in water tanks.

Economics

40. Perform a whole-life costing analysis and consider the following:
    - value of the net reduction in mains water supplied
    - value of the net reduction in wastewater discharge to the sewer system
    - total installed cost
    - cost of consumables including chemicals and power
    - cost of maintenance by site personnel or occupants
    - cost of maintenance by installer or maintenance company
    - lifetime and replacement cost of major parts.

32   RECLAIMED WATER SYSTEMS – GREYWATER

Project title... **Project No.**................................ **Design stage**...................

Engineer... **Revision No**................................ **Date**...............................

Checked by.. **Approved by**............................. **Date**...............................

Design inputs

- Patterns of water demand and use ☐
- Source and contamination levels of greywater ☐
- Likely volumes of water available for recycling ☐
- Quality and chemical composition of available water ☐

Notes / Design file cross-reference

Design outputs

- Size and location of storage tanks ☐
- Distribution pipework ☐
- Filtration and water treatment methodology ☐
- See Design Outputs for Reclaimed Water Systems - General ☐

Notes / Design file cross-reference

Key design checks

- Define potential greywater uses ☐
- Assess available water sources ☐
- Confirm that the greywater system is applicable for the application ☐
- Size the storage tank on a security of supply basis ☐
- Estimate costs and benefits ☐
- Maintenance access for the de-sludging of settlement tanks ☐

Notes / Design file cross-reference

Project specific checks and notes

☐
☐
☐

Notes / Design file cross-reference

32 RECLAIMED WATER SYSTEMS – GREYWATER

Design inputs

- Patterns of water demand and use
- Source and contamination levels of greywater
- Likely volumes of water available for recycling
- Quality and chemical composition of available water

Design information

- Required water treatment and disinfection
- Available space and location for storage tanks
- Available drainage
- Check acceptability with water authority

Design outputs

- Size and location of storage tanks
- Distribution pipework
- Filtration and water treatment methodology
- See Design Outputs for Reclaimed Water Systems - General

Key design checks

- Define potential greywater uses
- Assess available water sources
- Confirm that the greywater system is applicable for the application
- Size the storage tank on a security of supply basis
- Estimate costs and benefits
- Maintenance access for the de-sludging of settlement tanks

See also: Cold Water Storage Distribution, Legionnaires' Disease – Cold Water Services, Reclaimed Water Systems – General, Reclaimed Water Systems – Rainwater

Note: Reference must be to Reclaimed Water Systems - General

DESIGN WATCHPOINTS

Sizing and selection

1. Check that the design incorporates a method of greywater disinfection to counter the probable presence of pathogenic microorganisms. Choose between chemical disinfection, UV disinfection, and biological treatment or reed beds.

2. If chlorine-based disinfectants are to be used, check that this will be applied after any polymeric-membrane filter systems.

3. When disinfection is to be used, check that the disinfectant is actively mixed throughout the greywater, and that reliance is not placed on diffusion.

4. Check that the system will prevent untreated greywater entering the supply if the disinfectant runs out.

5. Check that the system can cope with the worst conceivable contamination from known sources.

6. Check that the storage capacity is not oversized. Check that greywater is not stored for more than 24 h untreated and more than three days after treatment.

7. Provide a manual way of draining greywater in response to exceptionally heavy loadings.

8. Ensure that greywater is filtered prior to treatment and storage. Consider the use of self-cleaning filters as these reduce the reliance on user intervention and reduce pump wear.

9. Check that UV disinfection is only used where the reclaimed water has a low turbidity and a low biological oxygen demand. Note that UV disinfection is not recommended as a primary treatment method for greywater.

10. Check that all faecally contaminated waste water (black water), such as that from WC's and bidets is designed to pass directly into the sewer system.

11. Check that dedicated greywater stacks and supply pipework can be accommodated within the space allocated for services.

Installation, operation and control

12. Check that greywater irrigation is not used for crops intended for eating. Greywater irrigation is not generally recommended; however, if applied its use should be restricted to sub-surface irrigation, such as tree and shrub watering.

13. Check that the operational status of the system will be clearly indicated to the user. This should include when disinfection top-up is required.

14. Check that an appropriate user manual is prepared. This should include details of:
    - emergency isolation procedure
    - start up and shutdown procedures
    - procedures to be followed in response to a faecal incident or heavily soiled greywater
    - response procedures relating to system alarms
    - required maintenance tasks and procedures
    - where to obtain consumables
    - and where to obtain advice.

15. When estimating greywater availability, consider the amount of water required for back-washing of filters, system drain downs following periods of non-use, along with manual diversion of greywater for tank cleaning or when greywater is too heavily contaminated.

16. Where necessary, check that adequate provision will be provided to connect and monitor through the building management system.

Access and maintenance

17. To allow for internal inspection and testing, check that the system can be emptied to the foul sewer using a manually operated valve.

18. Check that a bypass to sewer arrangement is installed to allow easy cleaning and maintenance following a faecal contamination.

19. Include a detailed building log book with maintenance activities.

Economics

20. Consider that maintenance, disinfection and electricity costs can outweigh the potential savings from reduced consumption of mains water.

21. Consider that greywater systems are more suited to new build applications than retrofit. For the latter, existing drainage systems must be modified and new pipework routed through the existing building.

22. Carry out life-cycle cost appraisal.

33 RECLAIMED WATER SYSTEMS – RAINWATER

Project title .... **Project No** .... **Design stage** ....

Engineer .... **Revision No** .... **Date** ....

Checked by .... **Approved by** .... **Date** ....

Design inputs

- Rainfall data
- Proposed catchment area
- Potential rainwater uses and demand, and associated required water quality

Notes / Design file cross-reference

Design outputs

- Size and location of storage tank(s)
- Filtration and water treatment methodology
- Optimum water storage period to cater for a likely drought period without oversizing the tank
- See Design Outputs for Reclaimed Water Systems - General

Notes / Design file cross-reference

Key design checks

- Water treatment requirements
- Optimum size of water storage tank(s)
- Material options for tanks and components

Notes / Design file cross-reference

Project specific checks and notes

Notes / Design file cross-reference

33 RECLAIMED WATER SYSTEMS – RAINWATER

Design inputs

- Rainfall data
- Proposed catchment area
- Potential rainwater uses and demand, and associated required water quality

Design information

- Potential location for storage tank(s)
- Catchment area material and slope
- Type and condition of existing catchment surfaces
- Check acceptability with the water authority

Design outputs

- Size and location of storage tank(s)
- Filtration and water treatment methodology
- Optimum water storage period to cater for a likely drought period without oversizing the tank
- See Design Outputs for Reclaimed Water Systems - General

Key design checks

- Water treatment requirements
- Optimum size of water storage tank(s)
- Material options for tanks and components

See also: Cold Water Storage and Distribution, Legionnaires' Disease – Cold Water Services, Roof Drainage, Reclaimed Water Systems – General, Reclaimed Water Systems – Greywater

Note: Reference must be made to Reclaimed Water Systems - General

DESIGN WATCHPOINTS

Sizing and selection

1. Select between indirectly-pumped systems, directly pumped systems, and gravity fed systems.

2. Check that an appropriate run-off coefficient has been used when determining the amount of water that can be harvested. The run-off coefficient reflects the collection surface material and pitch and takes into account instances of brief rainfall where there is insufficient water to enter the storage tank.

3. Consider that water harvested from areas such as pavements, roads and car parks will require treatment to remove animal faeces, grit, plant debris and oils. Water harvested from roofs will be contaminated by leaves, dust and grit, and bird droppings.

4. Consider that roof materials will affect the quality of harvested water, uncoated copper, lead and zinc roofs result in higher concentrations of metals in the water. Lead, rusted galvanised roofing sheet and zinc roofs must be avoided where the harvested water is to be used for potable use as the levels of contamination could exceed drinking water standards.

5. Consider that moss acts as a source of bacterial contamination. Consider the use of non-retentive roof surfaces that reduce moss and growth of algae.

6. Check that the gradient of gutters is sufficient to ensure that ponding does not occur. Consider the use of gutter guards to keep the gutters free of large debris. (Note that during heavy rain, water may flow over the guard, hence reducing water collection efficiency.)

7. When sizing the storage tank (or other form of facility) consider the following factors: catchment areas, rainfall pattern, demand pattern, retention time (time water will be stored in the tank), component costs, and costs and availability of alternative supplies.

8. Check that the selected tank is sufficiently large so that it does not frequently overflow, but is not so large that it causes stagnation.

9. To maintain beneficial biological activity, check the tank design to ensure that the feed inlet is at the bottom of the storage tank but above the likely level of sediment.

10. Check that an appropriate means of filtration is installed upstream of the collection tank. Consider the use of filters that do not require cleaning, such as self-cleaning downpipe filters and vortex filters.

11. Check that an appropriate means of filtration is installed to filter the water from the collection tank, such as floating filters, cartridge filters, slow sand filters, rapid gravity filters, membrane filters, and activated carbon filters.

12. Consider the use of biological treatment, such as reed beds.

13. Check whether water disinfection is required. Appropriate means of disinfection include ultra-violet systems and chemical disinfection. Disinfection is not required where rainwater from a catchment area with low contamination is used for toilet flushing, washing machines and irrigation, and where the system is well designed and operated.

14. Check that the water will be sufficiently filtered prior to the disinfection process.

15. Consider that porous pavements can be used to reduce containment of harvested water and as a first level of treatment.

16. Check that a mains water back-up supply is provided.

17. Consider the use of an above ground pump as opposed to a submersible pump to reduce tank access requirements.

18. Check compatibility between component parts to ensure no bimetallic corrosion.

Installation, operation and control

19. Check that rainwater is stored in the dark to prevent algal growth.

20. Check that tanks are vented to prevent the build up of harmful and potentially harmful gases.

21. Check that controls fail-safe to give mains water supply during power failure (or drought conditions), otherwise the water supply to outlets will fail.

22. Where necessary check that adequate provision will be provided to connect and monitor through the building management system.

Access and maintenance

23. Note that the regular cleaning of catchment areas and gutters will significantly reduce the risk of contamination.

24. Include a building log book noting components and trigger for maintenance activities.

Economics

25. Carry out a life-cycle cost appraisal, as the sizing of collection tanks requires careful evaluation.

26. The use of UV and chemical disinfection will increase operating costs.

27. Disposal filters will increase running costs compared to self-maintaining filters.

28. Pumping costs are a significant part of overall running costs.

29. Check for availability of government grants or tax incentives.

34   PIPED SERVICES

Project title .... **Project No.** .... **Design stage** ....

Engineer .... **Revision No** .... **Date** ....

Checked by .... **Approved by** .... **Date** ....

Design inputs

- Operating pressure ☐

- Required flowrate ☐

- Maximum permissible pressure-drop ☐

- Any allowable diversity of demand ☐

✓ **Notes / Design file cross-reference**

Design outputs

- Size of piping and material, insulation and lagging and pipe identification ☐

- Requirement for ancillary devices ☐

- Plant sizing, such as compressed air plant, vacuum plant, bulk oxygen vacuum-insulated evaporator (VIE) units, gas manifold rooms, liquid petroleum gas (LPG) storage tanks ☐

- Position of any medical gas isolating valves (area valve service units) ☐

✓ **Notes / Design file cross-reference**

Key design checks

- Where appropriate, check for compliance with *Pressure Systems Safety Regulation 2000* and associated approved codes of practice ☐

✓ **Notes / Design file cross-reference**

Project specific checks and notes

☐
☐
☐

✓ **Notes / Design file cross-reference**

34 PIPED SERVICES

Design inputs

- Operating pressure
- Required flowrate
- Maximum permissible pressure-drop
- Any allowable diversity of demand

Design information

- Piped services required
- Terminal outlet locations
- Plant locations
- Consumption figures for bottled and bulk liquid gases

Design outputs

- Size of piping and its material, insulation and lagging and pipe identification
- Requirement for ancillary devices
- Plant sizing, such as compressed air plant, vacuum plant, bulk oxygen vacuum-insulated evaporator (VIE) units, gas manifold rooms, liquid petroleum gas (LPG) storage tanks
- Position of any medical gas isolating valves (area valve service units)

Key design checks

- Where appropriate, check for compliance with *Pressure Systems Safety Regulation 2000* and associated approved codes of practice

---

DESIGN WATCHPOINTS

Gas fuels

1. Design and install gas installations in accordance with *IGE/UP/2 Gas Installation of Pipework, Boosters and Compressors on Industrial and Commercial Premises* and *CORGI's Essential Gas Safety*.

2. Check the availability, supply pressure and safety requirements of any proposed gas supply. Consider the requirements for future extension.

3. Inform the gas supplier if a gas compressor is to be used.

4. Check that pipes, fittings and components comply with British Standards.

5. Size the gas pipework in accordance with Section 11.1.3 of *CIBSE Guide G*.

6. Consider the requirement for filters.

7. For buried piping, follow the recommendations of Section 11.1.4.2 of *CIBSE Guide G*.

8. For piping in ducts or above ground follow the recommendations of Section 11.1.4.3 of *CIBSE Guide G*.

9. For gas boosters follow the recommendations of Section 11.1.5 of *CIBSE Guide G*.

10. For liquid petroleum gas installations check that the system is designed and installed in accordance with the *LP Gas Association Code of Practice 22*.

Non-medical compressed air

11. Check that the system is designed and installed in accordance with the *British Compressed Air Society Installation Guide*.

12. Check that the system complies with *BS ISO 4414*.

Medical compressed air

13. Check that the system is designed and installed in accordance with *NHS Estates' HTM 2022*.

Medical vacuum

14. Check that the system is designed and installed in accordance with *NHS Estates' HTM 2022*.

Medical gases

15. Check that the system is designed and installed in accordance with the following:
    - HTM 2022
    - BS 5682
    - BS EN 737
    - BS EN 739
    - CP23 (British Compressed Gas Association).

Economics

16. Perform a cost appraisal of installation options for alternative connection and fixing systems and the potential need for future adaptability.

35   FIRE SYSTEMS – WATER SUPPLY

Project title.. **Project No**................................. **Design stage**..................

Engineer.. **Revision No** .... **Date**................................

Checked by .... **Approved by** .... **Date** ....

Design inputs

- Flow rate and pressure of available mains water ☐

- Height of building ☐

- The required quantity of water for fire hydrants, and dry and wet risers, and to meet the requirements of the Fire Brigade ☐

- Number and location of required hose reels ☐

- Availability of duplicate water supplies ☐

Notes / Design file cross-reference

Design outputs

- Size of water supply pipes ☐

- Arrangements for providing appropriate flow rates and pressure ☐

Notes / Design file cross-reference

Key design checks

- Requirement for fire services water supplies. Check for design in accordance with *BS 5306-1* ☐

- Requirement for water supply for hose reels ☐

- Requirement for water supply for sprinklers. Check for design in accordance with the Loss Prevention Council's *Rules for Automatic Sprinkler Installation* ☐

Notes / Design file cross-reference

Project specific checks and notes

☐
☐
☐

Notes / Design file cross-reference

© BSRIA BG2/2006

35   FIRE SYSTEMS – WATER SUPPLY

Design inputs

- Flow rate and pressure of available mains water
- Height of building
- The required quantity of water for fire hydrants, and dry and wet risers, and to meet the requirements of the Fire Brigade
- Number and location of required hose reels
- Availability of duplicate water supplies

Design information

- Analysis of the local water supply for its potential to cause corrosion
- Type of fire systems to be installed that require a water supply
- Type of rising mains
- Hazard classification of building or area to be protected
- Required classification of water supply for sprinklers
- Hydrant locations

Design outputs

- Size of water supply pipes
- Arrangements for providing appropriate flow rates and pressure

Key design checks

- Requirement for fire services water supplies. Check for design in accordance with *BS 5306-1*
- Requirement for water supply for hose reels
- Requirement for water supply for sprinklers. Check for design in accordance with the Loss Prevention Council's *Rules for Automatic Sprinkler Installation*

See also: Mains Water Availability

DESIGN WATCHPOINTS

Sizing and selection – Fire services water supplies

1. Check with the water undertaker or supply company that sufficient quantities of water will be available.
2. Determine the requirement for fire hydrants. Check that sufficient flow for large jets will be available.
3. Check whether the use of fire tanks or open water sources will be required.
4. Check which type of fire mains will be most appropriate: dry rising mains, wet rising mains or charged dry rising mains.
5. Check that dry rising mains will be designed in accordance with Part 1 of BS 5306.
6. Check that charged dry rising mains comply with Parts 2,3,4 and 5 of BS 5041 and BS 5306 Part 1 with the addition of a header tank. Confirm the required size of the tank (typically 300 litres) with the fire authority.

Sizing and selection – Hose reels

7. Check that the water supply will provide a minimum flow of 30 l/min at the nozzle while sustaining simultaneous operation of two reels in the most hydraulically unfavourable positions.
8. Check that the length of the jet will be approximately 6 m at the minimum delivery rate.
9. Check with the hose reel manufacturer what is the required operating inlet pressure.
10. Select the most appropriate means of water supply:
    - direct from the mains water supply
    - using booster pumps on the mains water supply (where permitted)
    - or by pumping from a suction tank.
11. Check that there will be a dedicated hose reel water supply throughout the building.
12. Where a pumped system is to be used, check that duplicate pumps will be provided (duty and standby) with automatic activation on pressure or flow drop. Consider the use of a packaged hose reel pump.
13. Where a suction tank is to be used, check that the tank will have a minimum capacity of 1125 litres with automatic infill from the main supply via a pipe with a minimum diameter of 50 mm.
14. Check that the pipework is sized correctly to provide the required flows and pressures at the hose reel nozzles.

Sizing and selection – Sprinklers

15. Check the hazard classification: light hazard, ordinary hazard, or high hazard.
16. Check that the arrangements for water supply meets the requirements of the Loss Prevention Council's *Rules for Automatic Sprinkler Installation* (Note that the rules incorporate BS EN 12845).
17. Consider the requirement for reliability of water supplies. Check which is the most appropriate: single supply, superior supply, or duplicate supply. Note that any of these is appropriate for light or ordinary hazard risks. High hazard risks will require superior or duplicate supplies.
18. Check that mains water can provide adequate water supply. Check for any likely or possible future changes.
19. Check that the design capacity of the tanks is adequate.
20. Check that power supplies to pumps will be maintained at all times.
21. Check that where duplicate pumps are to be specified each pump can meet the required duty.
22. Check whether the sprinkler system has to be subdivided into sections. Check that separate pumps or pump stages are specified for each section.
23. Check that pipes are sized correctly.
24. Check that suitable control and alarm features are specified.

Installation, operation and control

25. Check that pipes will not be subjected to frost conditions. Provide insulation/trace heating where appropriate.

© BSRIA BG2/2006

DESIGN CHECKS – BIBLIOGRAPHY

Whole life costing

CIBSE *Guide to Ownership, Operation and Maintenance of Building Services*. 2000. ISBN 1 90328705 7

BLP Construction Durability Database – www.component life.com. (Data includes component durability, maintenance requirements and frequencies, component failure modes and causes and key durability issues)

Health and safety

HSC. *Managing Health and Safety in Construction. Construction (Design and Management) Regulations 1994*. Approved Code of practice and guidance. 2002. ISBN 0 7176 2139 1

HSE. Construction Information Sheet No 41. *Construction (Design and Management) Regulations 1994: The role of the designer*

HSE. *Control of Substances Hazardous to Health. The Control of Substances Hazardous to Health Regulations 2002*. Approved code of practice and guidance L5. 2002. ISBN 0 7176 2737 3

HSE. *Safe Work in Confined Spaces. Confined Spaces Regulations 1997*. Approved code of practice, regulations and guidance L101. 1997. ISBN 0 7176 1405 0

HSC. L8: *The control of Legionella Bacteria in Water Systems*. Approved Code of practice and guidance. HSE 2000. ISBN 07176 17726

The Stationary Office. *Work at Height Regulations 2005*. SI 2005/735

HSE. *The Work at Height Regulations 2005*. INDG401. A brief guide. 2005

Safe Use of Work Equipment. Provision and Use of Work Equipment Regulations 1998. Approved code of practice and guidance. L22. 2001. ISBN 0 7176 1626 6

Water Regulations Advisory Scheme. Water regulations guide. WRAS 2000. ISBN 09539708 0 09

Local authority requirements and discharge contents

Approved Document H – Drainage and Waste Disposal

BS EN 12056-5:2000. Gravity drainage systems inside buildings

BS EN 752 (Parts 1 to 7). Drain and sewer systems outside buildings

BS EN 1610 –1998 Construction and testing of drains and sewers

Sewers for Adoption Fifth edition. WRc 2001. ISBN 1 898920 43 5

Environment Agency *Pollution Prevention Guidelines* – PPG 1 *General Guide to Prevention of Pollution*, PPG 3 *Use and Design of Oil Separators in Surface Water Drainage Systems*

CIBSE, *Guide G: Public Health Engineering*. CIBSE 2004. ISBN 1 903287 42 1

The Institute of Plumbing. *Plumbing Engineering Services Design Guide*. The Institute of Plumbing 2002. ISBN 1 871956 40 4 (Now known as The Institute of Plumbing and Heating Engineering)

Mains water availability

Water Regulations Advisory Scheme. *Water Regulations Guide*. Water Regulations Advisory Scheme 2000. ISBN 0 953970 80 9

BS 6700:1997. Specification for design, installation, testing and maintenance of services supplying water for domestic use within buildings and their curtilages. ISBN 0 580 26817 9

BS EN 806-2:2005. Specification for installations inside buildings conveying water for human consumption. Part 2: Design

CIBSE, *Guide G: Public Health Engineering*. CIBSE 2004. ISBN 1 903287 42 1

The Institute of Plumbing. *Plumbing Engineering Services Design Guide*. The Institute of Plumbing 2002. ISBN 1 871956 40 4. Now known as The Institute of Plumbing and Heating Engineering

HSC, L8: *The Control of Legionella Bacteria in Water Systems*. Approved code of practice and guidance. HSE 2000. ISBN 0 7176 1772 6

Contamination prevention

Water Regulations Advisory Scheme. *Water Regulations Guide*. WRAS. 2000. ISBN 09539708-0-9

BS 6700:1997. Specification for design, installation, testing and maintenance of services supplying water for domestic use within buildings and their curtilages. ISBN 0 580 26817 9

BS EN 806-2:2005. Specification for installations inside buildings conveying water for human consumption. Part 2: Design

BS 1710:1984: Specification for identification of pipelines and services

BS EN 1717:2001. Protection against pollution of potable water in water installations and general requirements of devices to prevent pollution by backflow

The Institute of Plumbing. *Plumbing Engineering Services Design Guide*. 2002. ISBN 1 871956 40 4. (Now known as The Institute of Plumbing and Heating Engineering.)

Water conservation

BS 6700:1997. Specification for design, installation testing and maintenance of services supplying water for domestic use within buildings and their curtilages. ISBN 0 580 26817 9

BS EN 806-2:2005. Specification for installations inside buildings conveying water for human consumption. Part 2: Design

Water Regulations Advisory Scheme. *Water Regulations Guide*. WRAS. 2000. ISBN 09539708-0-9

Hot and Cold Water Supply. R H Garrett. 2000. ISBN 0-632-04985-5

The Institute of Plumbing. *Plumbing Engineering Services Design Guide*. 2002. ISBN 1 871956 40 4. (Now known as The Institute of Plumbing and Heating Engineering.)

Pipe sizing cold and hot water services

BS 6700:1997. Specification for design, installation, testing and maintenance of services supplying water for domestic use within buildings and their curtilages. ISBN 0 580 26817 9

BS EN 806-2:2005. Specification for installations inside buildings conveying water for human consumption. Part 2: Design

CIBSE, *Guide G: Public Health Engineering*. CIBSE 2004. ISBN 1 903287 42 1

CIBSE, *Guide C: Reference Data*. CIBSE 2001. ISBN 0750653604

The Institute of Plumbing. *Plumbing Engineering Services Design Guide*. The Institute of Plumbing 2002. ISBN 1 871956 40 4 (Now known as the Institute of Plumbing and Heating Engineering.)

© BSRIA BG2/2006

DESIGN CHECKS – BIBLIOGRAPHY

Pipe sizing above ground sanitary pipework
BS EN 12056-2:2000. Gravity drainage systems inside buildings – Part 2: Sanitary pipework, layout and calculation

BS EN 12109:1999. Vacuum drainage systems inside buildings

Approved Document H. Drainage and Waste Disposal. H1 Foul Water Drainage. TSO 2002. ISBN 0 11 753607 5

CIBSE, Guide G: Public Health Engineering. CIBSE 2004. ISBN 1 903287 42 1

The Institute of Plumbing. *Plumbing Engineering Services Design Guide.* 2002. ISBN 1 871956 40 4. (Now known as The Institute of Plumbing and Heating Engineering.)

Foul water below ground, drainage system sizing
Approved Document H. Drainage and Waste Disposal. H1 Foul Water Drainage. TSO 2002. ISBN 0 11 753607 5

BS EN 12056-2. Gravity drainage systems inside buildings. Part 2 Sanitary pipework, layout and calculation

CIBSE, Guide G: Public Health Engineering. CIBSE 2004. ISBN 1 903287 42 1

BS EN 752-4: 1998 Drain and sewer systems outside buildings. Hydraulic design and environmental considerations

Cold water storage and distribution
Water Regulations Advisory Scheme. *Water Regulations Guide.* Water Regulations Advisory Scheme 2000. ISBN 0 953970 80 9

Water Regulations Advisory Scheme. *Information and Guidance Note 9-04-04*, December 2003. Cold water storage cisterns – Design recommendations for mains supply inlets

BS 6700:1997. Specification for design, installation, testing and maintenance of services supplying water for domestic use within buildings and their curtilages. ISBN 0 580 26817 9

BS EN 806-2:2005. Specification for installations inside buildings conveying water for human consumption. Part 2: Design

BS 1710:1984. Specification for identification of pipelines and services

BS 7671:2001. Requirements for electrical installations (also known as the IEE Wiring Regulations)

BS 8313:1997. Code of practice for accommodation of building services in ducts

CIBSE, Guide G: Public Health Engineering. CIBSE 2004. ISBN 1 903287 42 1

CIBSE, Commissioning Code W. Water Distribution Systems. 2003. ISBN 1903287391

BSRIA AG 2/89.3. Commissioning Water Systems in Buildings. 2002. ISBN 086022 584 4

The Institute of Plumbing. *Plumbing Engineering Services Design Guide.* The Institute of Plumbing 2002. ISBN 1 871956 40 4. (Now known as The Institute of Plumbing and Heating Engineering.)

BS 6465-1:1994. Sanitary installations. Code of practice for scale of provision, selection and installation of sanitary appliances

CIBSE, Guide to Ownership, Operation and Maintenance of Building Services. CIBSE 2000. ISBN 190328 705 7

NHS Estates. HTM2027. *Hot and Cold Water Supply Storage and Mains Services.* 1995

Water Regulation Advisory Scheme. *Water Fittings and Materials Directory*

Hot water storage and distribution
Water Regulations Advisory Scheme. *Water Regulations Guide.* Water Regulations Advisory Scheme 2000. ISBN 0 953970 80 9

BS 6700:1997. Specification for design, installation, testing and maintenance of services supplying water for domestic use within buildings and their curtilages. ISBN 0 580 26817 9

BS EN 806-2:2005. Specification for installations inside buildings conveying water for human consumption. Part 2: Design

BS 1710:1984. Specification for identification of pipelines and services

BS 8313:1997. Code of practice for accommodation of building services in ducts

CIBSE, Guide G: Public Health Engineering. CIBSE 2004. ISBN 1 903287 42 1

The Institute of Plumbing. *Plumbing Engineering Services Design Guide.* The Institute of Plumbing 2002. ISBN 1 871956 40 4. (Now known as The Institute of Plumbing and Heating Engineering.)

Building Regulations 2000. Approved Document G3: Hygiene – Hot Water Storage

HSC, L8: *The Control of Legionella Bacteria in Water Systems.* Approved code of practice and guidance. HSE 2000. ISBN 0 7176 1772 6

CIBSE, Commissioning Code W. Water Distribution Systems. 2003. ISBN 1903287391

BSRIA AG 2/89.3. Commissioning Water Systems in Buildings. 2002. ISBN 086022 584 4

NHS Estates. HTM2027. *Hot and Cold Water Supply Storage and Mains Services.* 1995

Water Regulation Advisory Scheme. *Water Fittings and Materials Directory*

Legionnaires disease – cold water services
CIBSE, TM 13: Minimising the Risk of Legionnaires' Disease - Section 5: Hot and Cold Water Services. CIBSE 2002. ISBN 1 903287 23 5

HSC, L8: *The Control of Legionella Bacteria in Water Systems. Approved Code of Practice and Guidance.* HSE 2000. ISBN 0 7176 1772 6

CIBSE, Guide G: Public Health Engineering. CIBSE 2004. ISBN 1 903287 42 1

The Institute of Plumbing. *Plumbing Engineering Services Design Guide.* The Institute of Plumbing 2002. ISBN 1 871956 40 4. (Now known as The Institute of Plumbing and Heating Engineering)

CIBSE, Guide G: Public Health Engineering. CIBSE 2004. ISBN 1 903287 42 1

The Institute of Plumbing. *Plumbing Engineering Services Design Guide.* The Institute of Plumbing 2002. ISBN 1 871956 40 4. (Now known as The Institute of Plumbing and Heating Engineering)

Water Regulations Advisory Scheme. *Water Regulations Guide.* Water Regulations Advisory Scheme 2000. ISBN 0 953970 80 9

DESIGN CHECKS – BIBLIOGRAPHY

Water Regulations Advisory Scheme. *Water Fittings and Materials Directory*

BS 6700:1997. *Specification for design, installation, testing and maintenance of services supplying water for domestic use within buildings and their curtilages.* ISBN 0 580 26817 9

BS 1710:1984. *Specification for identification of pipelines and services*

BSRIA AG 19/00. *Guide to Legionellosis – Operation and Maintenance.* 2000. ISBN 0 86022 547 X

BSRIA AG 21/00. *Legionellosis Control Log Book. 2000.* ISBN 0 86022 562 3

BSRIA AG 20/00. *Guide to Legionellosis – Risk Assessment.* 2000. ISBN 0 86022 561 5

BSRIA AG 4/94. *Guide to Legionellosis – Temperature Measurements for Hot and Cold Water Services.* 1994. ISBN 0 86022 366 3

BSRIA TN 6/96. *Ionisation Water Treatment for Hot and Cold Water Services.* 1996. ISBN 0 86022 438 4

Legionnaires disease hot water services
CIBSE, TM 13: *Minimising the Risk of Legionnaires' Disease - Section 5: Hot and Cold Water Services.* CIBSE 2002. ISBN 1 903287 23 5

HSC, L8: *The control of Legionella Bacteria in Water Systems.* Approved code of practice and guidance. HSE 2000. ISBN 0 7176 1772 6

Water Regulations Advisory Scheme. *Water Regulations Guide.* Water Regulations Advisory Scheme 2000. ISBN 0 953970 80 9

Water Regulations Advisory Scheme. *Water Fittings and Materials Directory*

BS 6700:1997. *Specification for design, installation, testing and maintenance of services supplying water for domestic use within buildings and their curtilages.* ISBN 0 580 26817 9

BSRIA AG 19/00. *Guide to Legionellosis – Operation and Maintenance.* 2000. ISBN 0 86022 547 X

BSRIA AG 21/00. *Legionellosis control Log Book. 2000.* ISBN 0 86022 562 3

BSRIA AG 20/00. *Guide to Legionellosis – Risk Assessment.* 2000. ISBN 0 86022 561 5

BSRIA AG 4/94. *Guide to Legionellosis – Temperature Measurements for Hot and Cold Water Services.* 1994. ISBN 0 86022 366 3

BSRIA TN 6/96. *Ionisation Water Treatment for Hot and Cold Water Services.* 1996. ISBN 0 86022 438 4

Pressure boosting of water
Water Regulations Advisory Scheme. *Water Regulations Guide.* Water Regulations Advisory Scheme 2000. ISBN 0 953970 80 9

BS 6700:1997. *Specification for design, installation, testing and maintenance of services supplying water for domestic use within buildings and their curtilages.* ISBN 0 580 26817 9

BS EN 806-2:2005. *Specification for installations inside buildings conveying water for human consumption. Part 2: Design*

CIBSE, Guide G: *Public Health Engineering – Section 2.4.2: Boosted Water Systems.* CIBSE 2004. ISBN 1 903287 42 1

The Institute of plumbing. *Plumbing Engineering Services Design Guide.* 2002. ISBN 1 871956 40 4 (Now known as The Institute of Plumbing and Heating Engineering)

Drinking water systems
Water Regulations Advisory Scheme. *Water Regulations Guide.* Water Regulations Advisory Scheme 2000. ISBN 0 953970 80 9

BS 6700:1997. *Specification for design, installation, testing and maintenance of services supplying water for domestic use within buildings and their curtilages.* ISBN 0 580 26817 9

BS EN 806-2:2005. *Specification for installations inside buildings conveying water for human consumption. Part 2: Design*

CIBSE, Guide G: *Public Health Engineering – Section 2.4.3: Cold Water Storage.* CIBSE 2004. ISBN 1 903287 42 1

The Institute of Plumbing. *Plumbing Engineering Services Design Guide.* The Institute of Plumbing 2002. ISBN 1 871956 40 4 (Now known as The Institute of Plumbing and Heating Engineering)

Water treatment
BS 6700:1997. *Specification for design, installation, testing and maintenance of services supplying water for domestic use within buildings and their curtilages.* ISBN 0 580 26817 9

BS EN 806-2:2005. *Specification for installations inside buildings conveying water for human consumption. Part 2: Design*

BS EN 13451-3:2001. *Swimming pool equipment – Part 3: Additional specific safety requirements and test methods for pool fittings for water treatment purposes.* ISBN 0 580 37464 5

Water Regulations Advisory Scheme. *Water Regulations Guide.* WRAS. 2000. ISBN 09539708-0-9

HSC. L8: *The Control of Legionella Bacteria in Water System.* Approved Code of Practice and Guidance. HSE 2000. ISBN 0 7176 1772 6

CIBSE. Guide G: *Public Health Engineering.* CIBSE 2004. ISBN 1 903287 42 1

Pool Water Treatment Advisory Group (PWTAG). *Swimming Pool Water Treatment and Quality Standards.* 1999

BS 8300:2001. *Design of buildings and their approaches to meet the needs of disabled people – Code of practice.* ISBN 0 580 38438 1

Sanitary accommodation requirements
Approved Document G1 – *Sanitary Conveniences and Washing Facilities*

Approved Document M – *Access to and Use of Buildings*

Approved Document F – *Ventilation*

BS 6465-1:1994. *Sanitary installations. Part 1. Code of practice for scale of provision, selection and installation of sanitary appliances.* ISBN 0 580 23275 1

BS 6465-2:1996. *Sanitary installations. Part 2. Code of practice for space requirements for sanitary appliances.* ISBN 0 580 25456 9

BS 8300:2001. *Design of buildings and their approaches to meet the needs of disabled people – Code of practice.* ISBN 0 580 38438 1

The Institute of Plumbing. *Plumbing Engineering Services Design Guide.* The Institute of Plumbing 2002. ISBN 1 871956 40 4. (Now known as The Institute of Plumbing and Heating Engineering.)

CIBSE 2000. *Guide to Ownership, Operation and Maintenance of Building Services.* ISBN 190328 705 7

© BSRIA BG2/2006

DESIGN CHECKS – BIBLIOGRAPHY

Drainage systems, above ground foul drainage
Approved Document H – Drainage and Waste Disposal

BS EN 12056-5:2000. Gravity drainage systems inside buildings

BS EN 12109:1999. Vacuum drainage systems inside buildings

BS EN 476:1998. General requirements for components used in discharge pipes, drains and sewers for gravity systems

CIBSE, Guide G: Public Health Engineering. CIBSE 2004. ISBN 1 903287 42 1

CIBSE, Guide to Ownership, Operation and Maintenance of Building Services. CIBSE 2000. ISBN 1 903287057

The Institute of Plumbing. *Plumbing Engineering Services Design Guide.* The Institute of Plumbing 2002. ISBN 1 871956 40 4. (Now known as The Institute of Plumbing and Heating Engineering.)

Wise A F E, Swaffield J A 2002. *Water, Sanitary Waste Services for Buildings,* Fifth edition. Butterworth Heinemann. ISBN 0 7506 5255 1

BLP Construction Durability Database – www.componentlife .com (lists durability factors for above ground drainage components)

Ministry of Defence. Defence Estates Organisation (Works). *Space Requirements for Plant Access, Operation and Maintenance. Design and Maintenance Guide 8.* ISBN 0117727857

Foul water, below ground drainage systems
Approved Document H. Drainage and Waste Disposal. TSO 2002. ISBN 0 11 753607 5

BS EN 752 (Parts 1 to 7). Drain and sewer systems outside buildings

BS EN 1295-1:1998. Structural design of buried pipelines under various conditions of loading

BS EN 1610:1998. Construction and testing of drains and sewers

BS EN 12050 (Parts 1 to 4). Wastewater lifting plants for buildings and sites. Principles of construction and testing

BS EN 12056 (Parts 1 to 5). Gravity drainage systems inside buildings

BS EN 13564 (Parts 1 to 3). Anti-flooding devices in buildings

CIBSE, Guide G: Public Health Engineering. CIBSE 2004. ISBN 1 903287 42 1

WRC. *Sewers for Adoption.* 5th edition. 2001. ISBN 1 898920 43 5

The Institute of Plumbing. *Plumbing Engineering Services Design Guide.* 2002. ISBN 1 871956 40 4. (Now known as The Institute of Plumbing and Heating Engineering.)

Commercial kitchen drainage
BS EN 1825-1. Installation for separation of grease. Part 1: Principles of design, performance and testing, marking and quality control

BS EN 1825-2:2002. Grease separators – Part 2: Selection of nominal size, installation, operation and maintenance

BS EN 12056-2:2000. Gravity drainage systems inside buildings – Part 2: Sanitary pipework, layout and calculation

The Institute of Plumbing. (Now known as the Institute of Plumbing and Heating Engineering). *Plumbing Engineering Services Design Guide.* The Institute of Plumbing 2002. ISBN 1 871956 40 4

CIBSE, Guide G: Public Health Engineering. CIBSE 2004. ISBN 1 903287 42 1

Approved Document H. Drainage and Waste Disposal. Part H1 – Foul water drainage. TSO 2002. ISBN 0 11 753607 5

Surface water, below ground drainage systems
Approved Document H. Drainage and Waste Disposal. H3 Rainwater Drainage. TSO 2002. ISBN 0 11 753607 5

CIBSE, Guide G: Public Health Engineering. CIBSE 2004. ISBN 1 903287 42 1

Building Research Establishment. *Soakaway Design. BRE Digest 365.* 1991. ISBN 0901090 31X

BS EN 752-4:1998. Drain and sewer systems outside buildings – Part 4: Hydraulic design and environmental considerations

Environment Agency. PPG3. *Use and Design of Oil Separators in Surface Water Drainage Systems*

WRC. *Sewers for Adoption.* 5th edition. ISBN 1 898920 43 5

The Institute of Plumbing. *Plumbing Engineering Services Design Guide.* 2002. ISBN 1 871956 40 4. (Now known as The Institute of Plumbing and Heating Engineering.)

CIRIA 529 (suds)

Roof drainage

BS EN 12056-1:2000. Gravity drainage systems inside buildings – General and performance requirements

BS EN 12056-3:2000. Gravity drainage systems inside buildings – Roof drainage, layout and calculation

BS EN 12056-5:2000. Gravity drainage systems inside buildings – Installation and testing, instructions for operation, maintenance and use

BS 3868: 1995. Specification for prefabricated drainage stack units in galvanised steel

BS EN 607:1996. Eaves gutters and fittings made from PVC-U. Definitions, requirements and testing

BS EN 612:1996. Eaves gutters and rainwater downpipes of metal sheet. Definitions, classifications and requirements

BLP Construction Durability Database – www.componentlife.com – for durability data on components

Sustainable urban drainage systems
CIRIA, C523. *Sustainable Urban Drainage Systems – Best Practice Manual.* CIRIA 2001. ISBN 0 86017 523 5

CIRIA, C522. *Sustainable Urban Drainage Systems – Design Manual for England and Wales.* CIRIA 2001. ISBN 0 86017 522 7

CIRIA, C609. *Sustainable Drainage Systems. Hydraulic, Structural and Water Quality Advice*

Environment Agency Framework for Sustainable Drainage. 2003. Draft for consultation document

H R Wallingford/CIRIA. 2004. *Drainage of Development Sites – A Guide.* ISBN 0 86017 900 1

DESIGN CHECKS – BIBLIOGRAPHY AND REFERENCES

Reclaimed water systems, general

BSRIA TN 6/2002. *Water Reclamation Guidance. Design and Construction of Systems Using Grey Water*. 2002. ISBN 0 86022 597 6

BSRIA TN 7/2002. *Water Reclamation Standard. Laboratory Testing of Systems Using Grey Water*. 2002. ISBN 0 86022 598 4

BS EN 752. *Drain and sewer systems outside buildings*

WRAS. *Reclaimed Water Systems*. Information about installing, modifying, or maintaining reclaimed water systems. Information and guidance note 9-02-04. 1999

CIRIA. Project report 80. *Rainwater and Greywater Use in Buildings – Decision Making for Water Conservation*. 2001. ISBN 0 86017 880 3

WRAS. *Marking and Identification of Pipework for Reclaimed (Greywater) Systems*. Information and guidance note 9-02-05. 1999

CIRIA C539. *Rainwater and Greywater Use in Buildings – Best Practice Guidance*. 2001. ISBN 0 86017 539 1

BLP Construction Durability Database – www.componentlife.com (durability data on components)

Reclaimed water systems, greywater

BSRIA TN 6/2002. *Water Reclamation Guidance. Design and Construction of Systems Using Grey Water*. 2002. ISBN 0 86022 597 6

BSRIA TN 7/2002. *Water Reclamation Standard. Laboratory Testing of Systems Using Grey Water*. 2002. ISBN 0 86022 598 4

WRAS. *Reclaimed Water Systems. Information About Installing, Modifying, or Maintaining Reclaimed Water Systems*. Information and guidance note 9-02-04. 1999

CIRIA. Project report 80. *Rainwater and Greywater Use in Buildings – Decision Making for Water Conservation*. 2001. ISBN 0 86017 880 3

WRAS. *Marking and Identification of Pipework for Reclaimed (Greywater) Systems*. Information and guidance note 9-02-05. 1999

CIRIA C539. *Rainwater and Greywater Use in Buildings – Best Practice Guidance*. 2001. ISBN 0 86017 539 1

BLP Construction Durability Database – www.componentlife.com (durability data on components)

Reclaimed water systems, rainwater

BSRIA TN 6/2002. *Water Reclamation Guidance. Design and Construction of Systems Using Grey Water*. 2002. ISBN 0 86022 597 6

BSRIA TN 7/2002. *Water Reclamation Standard. Laboratory Testing of Systems Using Grey Water*. 2002. ISBN 0 86022 598 4

WRAS. *Reclaimed Water Systems. Information About Installing, modifying, or Maintaining Reclaimed Water Systems*. Information and guidance note 9-02-04. 1999

CIRIA. Project report 80. *Rainwater and Greywater Use in Buildings – Decision Making for Water Conservation*. 2001. ISBN 0 86017 880 3

Water Regulations Advisory Scheme, WRAS. *Marking and Identification of Pipework for Reclaimed (Greywater) Systems*. Information and guidance note 9-02-05. 1999

CIRIA C539. *Rainwater and Greywater Use in Buildings – Best Practice Guidance*. 2001. ISBN 0 86017 539 1

See References/Bibliography for Roof Drainage

Piped services

Institution of Gas Engineers and Managers. IGE/UP/2. *Gas Installation of Pipework, Boosters and Compressors on Industrial and Commercial Premises*. 1994

CORGI. *Essential Gas Safety*, 2nd edition. 2001. ISBN 1-902632-00-1

CIBSE, Guide G: Public Health Engineering – Section 2.4.3: Cold Water Storage. CIBSE 2004. ISBN 1 903287 42 1

LP Gas Association. Code of Practice 22. *LPG Piping Systems – Design and Installation*. 2002

Health and Safety Commission. L122. *Safety of Pressure Systems. Pressure Systems Safety Regulation 2000*. Approved Code of practice. ISBN 0 7176 1767X

British Compressed Air Society. Installation Guide 5th edition. *Guide to the Selection and Installation of Compressed Air Services*. ISBN 0905608135

BS ISO 4414:1998, *Pneumatic fluid power. General rules relating to systems*

NHS Estates. HTM 2022. *Medical Gas Pipeline Systems. Design, Installation, Validation and Verification*. 1997. ISBN 0-11-322067-7

BS 5682:1998 *Specification for probes (quick connectors) for use with medical gas pipeline systems*

BS EN 737 *(Parts 1 to 4) Medical gas pipeline systems*

BS EN 739:1998 *Low-pressure hose assemblies for use with medical gases*

British Compressed Gas Association. CP 23. *Application of the Pressure Systems Safety Regulations 2000 to Industrial and Medical Pressure Systems Installed at User Premises*. 2002

Fire systems water supply

CIBSE Guide G. Public Health Engineering. 2004. ISBN 1 903287 42 1

CIBSE Guide E. Fire Engineering. 2003. ISBN 1903287316

BS 5041 *Fire hydrant systems equipment*
Part 1: 1987. *Specification for landing valves for wet risers*
Part 2: 1987. *Specification for landing valves for dry risers*
Part 3: 1975. *Specification for inlet breechings for dry riser inlets*
Part 4: 1975. *Specification for boxes for landing valves for dry risers*
Part 5: 1974. *Specification for boxes for foam inlets and dry riser inlets*

BS 5306 – 1:1976: *Fire extinguishing installations and equipment on premises. Hydrant systems, hose reels and foam inlets.*

LPC *Rules for automatic sprinkler Installations Incorporating BS EN 12845*. Fire Protection Association, ISBN 1-902790-25-1

REFERENCES

i. *BS EN ISO 9001:2000 Quality management systems – requirements* ISBN 0 580 36837 8
ii. *BS 7000 Pt4:1996 Guide to managing design in construction*
iii. Griffiths and Armour *Review of Claims Trends* 2004
iv. Griffiths and Armour : *The avoidance of Professional Indemnity Claims through Better Business Practice* 2005
v. *BS EN ISO 9004:2000 Quality management systems – Guidelines for performance improvements* ISBN 0 580 36838 6
vi. Cross N, *Design: Principles and Practice – Product Planning and the Design Brief*, Open University 1995 ISBN 07492 71892
vii. *ACE Conditions of Engagement Agreement A2, Appendix1, ACE 1998*
viii. EPSRC, IMI *Generic Design and Construction Process Protocol*

DESIGN CHECKS – GLOSSARY

Air admittance valve
Valve that allows air to enter a drainage system but not escape in order to limit pressure fluctuations within the sanitary pipework

Backflow
Flow of water in the opposite direction to that intended within or from a water fitting. Includes back-siphonage

Back-siphonage
Backflow caused by siphonage

Bedding
Material introduced around and under a pipe to improve its load resistance. Supports the pipe between the trench bottom and the sidefill or initial backfill

Black water
Waste water containing faecal matter or urine

Cistern
Tank used to store water at atmospheric pressure

Combined drainage system
System of drainage in which foul and surface water are conveyed in the same pipes to a common or combined sewer

Detention basin
Vegetated depression constructed to store water temporarily to attenuate flows

Discharge unit
Average discharge rate of a sanitary appliance expressed in litres per second

Drain
Near-horizontal pipe suspended within a building or buried in the ground to which stacks or ground floor appliances are connected

Filter drain
Drain consisting of a trench filled with permeable material

Filter strip
Gently sloping vegetated area that drains water off impermeable areas and filters out silt and other particles

Grease separator
Unit or assembly of units to separate grease from waste water and retain the separated grease within the unit

Grey water
Water originally supplied as wholesome water that has been used for bathing, washing, laundry or washing dishes

Infiltration basin
Dry basin designed to promote infiltration of surface water to the ground

Infiltration trench
Trench, usually filled with permeable granular material, designed to promote infiltration of surface water to the ground

Invert
Lowest point on the internal surface of a pipe or channel

Manhole
A chamber designed to enable access to the drain or sewer for inspection or maintenance

Potable water
Water that is suitable for human consumption (drinking water)

Reclaimed water
Water that has been treated so that its quality is suitable for particular specified purposes such as irrigation and toilet flushing

Retention pond
Pond where run-off is detained to allow settlement and possibly biological treatment of some pollutants

Return period
Occurrence frequency of an event, for example a return period of 10 years refers to a rate of rainfall that on average occurs once every 10 years

Run-off
Excess water that flows off the ground surface

Separate drainage system
System of drainage in which foul and surface water are segregated and discharged into separate sewers or other places of disposal

Soakaway
Pit, either unfilled and lined or filled with rubble, into which surface water is drained to infiltrate into the ground

Stack
Pipe (generally vertical) conveying discharges from sanitary appliances

Swale
Shallow, vegetated channel used to conduct and retain water. Can also allow infiltration

Trap
Device that prevents the passage of foul air by means of a water seal

Vacuum drainage
Transportation of waste water by vacuum. Makes use of the total head available between the outlets and the discharge point

Ventilating stack
Main vertical ventilating pipe, connected to a discharge stack, to limit pressure fluctuations within the discharge stack

Waste water
Waste water that is contaminated by use and all water discharging into a drainage system

Waste water lifting – plant
Device for the collection and automatic lifting of waste water to a height above flood level

Wetland
Pond that has a high proportion of emergent vegetation in relation to open water

Wholesome water
Water fit to drink. Fluid category 1 of the *Water Supply (Water Fittings) Regulations*

ALPHABETICAL LIST OF DESIGN CHECKS

© BSRIA BG2/2006

FEEDBACK FORM

BG 2/2006, *Design Checks for Public Health*

Please complete and return to:
Kevin Pennycook at BSRIA Ltd
Fax: 01344 465626

Page Number	Title	Comments

Name .... Email ....

Company ....

Address ....

....

.... Postcode ....

Telephone .... Fax ....

© BSRIA BG2/2006